The care of the human mind is the most noble branch of medicine.

Gaubius *On the Duty and Office of Physicians of the Mind*, c. 1750

At last somebody has defined the value of a psychiatrist. A man holding hostages at gunpoint at St. Jude Research Hospital, Memphis, released one of them—a psychiatrist—in return for five hamburgers, five cheeseburgers and some potato crisps.

The Times 8 February 1982

Rehabilitation in Psychiatry
An introductory handbook

Clephane Hume
Lecturer in Occupational Therapy,
Queen Margaret College, Edinburgh

Ian Pullen
Consultant Psychiatrist,
Royal Edinburgh Hospital;
Honorary Senior Lecturer,
University of Edinburgh

Churchill Livingstone ▦
EDINBURGH LONDON MELBOURNE AND NEW YORK 1986

CHURCHILL LIVINGSTONE
Medical Division of Longman Group Limited

Distributed in the United States of America by Churchill Livingstone Inc., 1560 Broadway, New York, N.Y. 10036, and by associated companies, branches and representatives throughout the world.

First published 1986

ISBN 0-443-02509-6

British Library Cataloguing in Publication Data
Rehabilitation in psychiatry.
  1. Mentally ill—Rehabilitation
  I. Hume, Clephane   II. Pullen, Ian
  362.2'0425   RC439.5

Library of Congress Cataloging in Publication Data
Hume, Clephane.
  Rehabilitation in psychiatry.
  1. Mentally ill—Rehabilitation.   2. Rehabilitation.
I. Pullen, Ian M.   II. Title.   [DNLM: 1. Mental
Disorders—rehabilitation.   WM 29.1 H921r]
RC439.5.H85   1986   616.89'16   85-11677

Produced by Longman Singapore Publishers (Pte) Ltd.
Printed in Singapore

Preface

Edinburgh has been called the 'Athens of the North' and, less charitably, the 'Reykjavik of the South'*. It is all a matter of perspective.

In many respects rehabilitation is in a similar position. What is called a 'rehabilitation unit' by one team may be described as a 'back ward' by another. In fact neither description is necessarily correct. This book attempts to set rehabilitation in perspective.

Many people will find themselves working in rehabilitation, either permanently or on placement, without any clear idea of what 'rehabilitation' means, its potential and its limitations. Others will be expected to know something about rehabilitation for examinations! Our intention has been to provide basic information in as readable a form as possible. The book should be short enough to be read from cover to cover (by the determined), but each chapter is written to be read on its own (for the selective).

While the book is written by members of different professions, we have tried to avoid the common pitfall of many multi-author books: that of presenting the doctor's, nurse's, occupational therapist's, psychologist's and social worker's

* Tom Stoppard 1972 *Jumpers* Faber, London, p. 69

views in turn. Most of the book has been written by two of us (an occupational therapist and a psychiatrist), but we invited clinical psychologists to write chapters on the psychological approach and on mental handicap. A nurse was invited to contribute a chapter on the multi-disciplinary team. The omission of a social worker reflects our wish to limit the number of contributors.

After an historical introduction we move to chapters describing the task of rehabilitation and the arguments for and against different treatment settings. Organisation and treatment planning follow, making a clear case for careful planning of all work with patients. The multi-disciplinary team has been reviewed critically with suggestions for improving teamwork. This chapter includes an important section on burnout—a particular risk in rehabilitation work.

Psychological approaches, the special problems of mental handicap and rehabilitation of the elderly and physically handicapped follow. We end with a brief look into the rehabilitation crystal ball.

For simplicity the pronoun 'he' is used throughout the book when referring to patients, staff or relatives. This convention has been followed as the English language has no single pronoun denoting both sexes, and s/he and he/she are unnecessarily clumsy.

We hope this book will be stimulating and thought-provoking, but the reader is warned that 'Reading is sometimes an ingenious device for avoiding thought'!**

This book has come through a long gestation period starting with encouragement from Dr James Affleck when we were both members of his rehabilitation team. It would not have seen the light of day without the support of our publisher Sally Morris, and the aciduous typing of Dianne Birse. We are grateful to all of them.

Edinburgh, 1986   C.H.
                                                                   I.P.

** Sir Arthur Helps 1847, 1853 *Friends in Council* Book 2, ch 1

Contributors

Jill Birrell
Senior Clinical Psychologist, Royal Edinburgh Hospital

Michael Henderson
Clinical Psychologist, Clifton Hospital, York. Formerly Clinical Psychologist, Royal Edinburgh Hospital

Clephane Hume
Lecturer in Occupational Therapy, Queen Margaret College, Edinburgh

Linda Pollock
Scottish Home and Health Department Research Fellow, Department of Nursing Studies, University of Edinburgh

Ian Pullen
Consultant Psychiatrist, Royal Edinburgh Hospital; Honorary Senior Lecturer, University of Edinburgh

Sheila Youngson
Senior Clinical Psychologist, Child and Adolescent Unit, Beck House, Scarborough. Formerly Senior Clinical Psychologist, Gogarburn Hospital, Edinburgh

Contents

The past is a foreign country: they do things differently there.

L.P. Hartley *The Go-Between*

1

Historical introduction

Ian Pullen

THE TURN OF A TIDE

Thirty years ago, a tide turned. For two centuries, the number of beds in Britain occupied by the mentally ill steadily increased. Then, in 1954, the peak was reached and numbers began to fall. At first, the fall was rapid, but after 1970 the trend continued at a slower pace. In the past 30 years, mental hospital beds have been reduced by a half.

This change has not been confined to Britain but has occurred throughout the West. In the United States, the peak hospital population was reached in 1955, since when numbers have fallen by two-thirds. Similar trends have been seen in Europe, Canada, Australia and New Zealand.

De-institutionalisation, the discharge of patients from hospital and their resettlement in the community, came about largely as a result of changing attitudes to care and was helped by the discovery and introduction of effective drugs. However, the major precipitant, both in Britain and the United States, was severe overcrowding in the large Victorian mental hospitals. The achievement of de-institutionalisation has not been without problems. There has been a huge increase in the number of admissions and readmissions to hospital, a higher turnover of patients and a rise in the number of discharged but disturbed former patients. Many of these ex-patients face bleak lives in doss-houses, bed and breakfast accommodation or common lodging houses. It is probably too early to say whether de-institutionalisation represents an 'enlightened revolution or an abdication of responsibility' (Bassuk and Gerson, 1978). Certainly we must ensure that we do not lose sight of what is best for an individual patient, rather than blindly follow the latest fashion.

BEGINNINGS

In medieval Britain, the poor and needy of all types, including the mentally disturbed, relied on the haphazard and rather ineffectual charity organised by the Church. Some of the mentally ill were left to wander as beggars while others relied on family or friends. In only a small minority of cases was any attempt made to relieve the family by gathering the ill together in institutions.

Bethlem, founded in 1247 as a Priory of the Order of St Mary of Bethlehem, took its first mental patient in 1377. Sited in London, it was the only public hospital in Britain for the care of the mentally ill until 1700. Its contribution was pitifully small. In 1403, it held six insane and three sane inmates. By 1632, there were 27 patients, and only towards the end of the 17th century did the number rise to 150.

The 17th and 18th centuries were times of great change. The dissolution of the monasteries and the confiscation of their lands put an end to much of the Church-based help. The population was rising rapidly at a time when changes in land use reduced the numbers required to work the land. The authorities, frightened by the 'army of vagrants and beggars', set up institutions (Bridewells) to confine a wide range of deviants including the mentally ill.

The growth of these institutions was interrupted in 17th century Britain by the Civil War, but on the continent continued apace—a period called the 'Great Confinement'.

THE GREAT CONFINEMENT

The Salpetrière, in Paris, was a classical example of the large, multi-purpose institution. In 1788 it was the largest hospital in France and possibly in Europe. It was a 'prison, a home for pregnant mothers and girls, wet-nurses, boys up to the age of 5, old people, the blind, epileptic, mad, and incurables of all sorts'.

In 18th-century Britain, the well-off mentally ill could be looked after in a variety of ways. They could be cared for in the home of a general physician or a clergyman, or could be confined in a Private Madhouse. These private madhouses were ordinary dwelling houses run for profit which began to spring up in the 1650s, reaching their peak in the early 19th century.

The poor (then known as paupers) had less choice. In the early part of the 18th century, the only hospital provision in Britain for the mentally ill remained the Bethlem in London and a newly opened hospital in Bristol. Many of the pauper insane were confined in Bridewells with criminals, vagrants and beggars.

From 1760 onwards, institutions became increasingly purpose-built as workhouses, prisons or hospitals, but only a handful of provincial towns established hospitals for the insane. The majority of 'pauper lunatics' began to be boarded out in private madhouses at the expense of the parish.

The rapid influx of the poor led to appalling overcrowding as private madhouse keepers found they could increase their income by taking more and more inmates. Another abuse of the private madhouse system was the occasional detention of the sane. Sometimes unscrupulous landlords would agree to lock up a sane person in return for a large fee. So wayward daughters or those about to gain an inheritance might conveniently be disposed of (there have been cases, even in this century, of the former.) The investigation of such cases revealed the dreadful conditions in which the insane were kept.

In 1774, for the first time, an Act of Parliament provided for the inspection and licensing of madhouses. The Act also introduced a form of *certification*. No person could be detained in a madhouse without the signature of a physician, a surgeon or an apothecary. So the beginning of mental health legislation was for the protection of the sane, to protect them from wrongful detention in conditions fit only for the insane. It was not directly to improve the lot of the insane (Jones, 1960). Much of the treatment of the day was physical and many were held under restraint by chains or straitjackets. There is no doubt that the madhouse keepers and physicians considered their treatment to be reasonable and carried out in the best interests of the patient. This description of the treatment of a Royal patient, George III, written at the time gives some flavour of those regimes:

'The unhappy patient . . . was no longer treated as a human being. His body was immediately encased in a machine which left no liberty for motion. He was sometimes chained to a stake. He was frequently beaten and starved, and at best, was kept in subjection by menacing and violent language.' (Scull, 1982)

The Protestant era, which began in the 17th century, emphasised the virtue of work, and thus condemned idleness, which led to the setting up of workhouses and houses of correction. But by the end of this period, things were beginning to change.

MORAL TREATMENT—THE BEGINNING OF REHABILITATION?

In 1793, Pinel was put in charge of the Bicêtre Asylum in Paris and quickly set about freeing patients from their chains. Tuke founded the Retreat Hospital in York and was one of the advocates of *moral treatment*. This was a general, pragmatic approach, making use of anything which appeared to work, with the aim of minimising external, physical coercion. Restraint might be necessary to prevent bodily injury but was the last resort. Tuke wrote that only by 'treating the patient as much in the manner of a rational being as the state of mind will allow' could one hope to re-educate him to discipline himself. He considered that the 'vital weapon' to be used in this re-education process was man's desire for esteem (Rosen, 1968).

The staff played a vital role in this process, treating patients with kindness and consideration. 'Whatever tends to promote the happiness of the patient, is found to increase his desire to restrain himself, by exciting the wish not to forfeit his enjoyments.' This use of rewards (we now call them re-inforcers) is very similar to modern behaviour modification techniques.

Occupation was recognised as being important. In 1801, Pinel wrote 'How pleasing to observe the silence and tranquillity which prevailed in the Bicêtre where nearly all the patients were supplied by tradesmen of Paris with employment which fixed their attention, and allured them to exertion by the prospect of trifling gain.'

The Retreat was a successful experiment and showed that an asylum could provide a comfortable and accepting environment. Writing in 1813, Tuke claimed that the statistics for the first 15 years of the Retreat showed that 'moral treatment could restore a large proportion of cases to sanity'. The asylum was to be a home where the patient could be known and treated as an individual, where his mind was to be constantly stimulated and encouraged to return to its natural state of health.

IDEAL AND REALITY

The 1808 County Asylum Act gave local magistrates power to provide asylums at the county's expense, but by 1830, only ten had opened. By 1845, as only a further eight had been built, a new Act made their provision mandatory. Progress seemed set to continue. In 1834 the small hospital at Lincoln abolished restraint and in 1839 John Connoly took the brave step of abolishing restraint in the 800 bed Hanwell Hospital.

But the rising population, the economic depression of the 1870s and a general change of philosophy caused a marked decline in the standard of care in these growing institutions. A select committee in 1859, investigating rumours of ill-treatment at Hanwell, commented on the major difficulty in recruiting staff of the right type. *The Times* in 1877 argued 'If lunacy continues to increase as at present, the insane will be in the majority and, freeing themselves, will put the sane in asylums'.

Further legislation followed. The 1890 Lunacy Act was long and complex. Counties were now compelled to build asylums and to tighten up on the admission procedures. Asylums were only to take certified patients and patients could not be certified until the illness had reached the stage where it was obvious.

THE TWENTIETH CENTURY

In the 1890s, asylum standards declined still further. The original idea had been for small institutions 'where the patient could be known', but by 1900, the average asylum contained 961 patients and by 1930, this number had risen to 1221. The barrack-like asylums had a different atmosphere and patients were treated *en masse*. Ten nurses dealing with 100 patients in a ward do not achieve the same quality of personal relationship as one nurse with ten patients. Patients worked on hospital farms and in the gardens but their work was organised for the maintenance of the institution, not for their own benefit. They moved from place to place in groups and were counted in and counted out of the wards by nurses who often could not remember their names or faces (Jones, 1960).

World War I brought a further reduction in standards as able-bodied staff were recruited to the Armed Forces. After the war conditions again began to improve: 1920 brought the opening of the Maudsley Hospital for voluntary patients, a change that required a special Act of Parliament.

In 1928, it was recommended that British mental hospitals should have someone similar to the almoners of the large voluntary general hospitals. Their job would be to 'allay the patients' anxieties about home conditions during treatment and to help with employment and any domestic difficulties after discharge'. The first British psychiatric social workers were American trained but in 1929 a training course was started at the London School of Economics.

The Royal Commission (1924–6), suggested that a special officer should be appointed in each hospital to direct patients' activities. In 1925, the first trained occupational therapist was employed in Aberdeen and more followed during the 1930s.

VOLUNTARY TREATMENT

The Mental Treatment Act, 1930, allowed for voluntary treatment: 'any person wishing of his own free will to undergo treatment could make a special application to the person in charge of the establishment'. However, a voluntary patient had to give 72 hours notice in writing if he wanted to discharge himself. The Act also gave local authorities the power to provide psychiatric out-patient facilities staffed by mental hospital doctors. Thus, these provisions supported by the growing Mental After Care Association allowed earlier treatment and follow-up.

The economic depression of the 30s brought about a doubling of unemployment to 20.8 per cent of the working population and fears that the unemployed might find life more comfortable as voluntary patients. But the situation also increased the number of staff available.

The period leading up to World War II saw moves to improve the environment in mental hospitals. By 1934 most hospitals held dances which broke down the rigid segregation of the sexes and the question of unlocked wards was being raised. At first, the introduction of open wards aroused anxieties but it was found that some very disturbed patients improved with the unlocking of doors.

The war brought the inevitable shortages and a return to locked doors because of low staffing levels. There was a fear that war would lower the threshhold for mental illness and in 1938 a committee of psychiatrists from London hospitals estimated that three to four million acute psychiatric cases could be expected within six months of the outbreak of war. By 1940 it was obvious that the estimates were wrong and that the bombing increased morale rather than lowered it.

THE NATIONAL HEALTH SERVICE

The immediate post-war period brought a change of government in Britain and the advent of the National Health Service as part of the welfare state. This was a period not only of administrative change but also of therapeutic development. In 1933 Insulin Coma Therapy brought the first successful treatment of severe depression. This was closely followed by Electro-Convulsive Therapy (E.C.T.) in 1938. Leucotomy (lobotomy), the surgical interruption of the nervous connections between the frontal lobes and the rest of the brain, was introduced in 1942. This treatment gained rapid popularity for the treatment of intractable psychosis and depression, reaching a peak in Britain in 1949 when 1200 leucotomoies were carried out, mainly for schizophrenia.

But it was not just physical methods of treatment that were innovative. The first British day hospital was opened in 1946 under the title 'Social Psychotherapy Centre', but was later renamed the Marlborough Day Hospital. A second day hospital was opened in Bristol five years later and by 1972 there were 12 600 day patients throughout Britain. In 1947 Maxwell Jones moved to the Henderson Hospital in London, taking with him the community and group methods that he had started during the war. The Henderson was the start of the *therapeutic community movement* which was to have so much influence on the running of mental hospitals and other institutions caring for people over succeeding decades.

The introduction of the National Health Service in Britain in 1948 allowed psychiatry to develop as a salaried medical service undiluted by the demands of private practice. Outpatient facilities were expanded; a variety of stepping-stones were placed between community and hospital, adding hostels to day hospitals. Domiciliary visits strengthened links with the general practitioner.

In the United States, on the other hand, the more usual way of providing psychiatric care was by office-based private practice. This allowed more intensive and prolonged psychotherapy to take place and consequently dynamic psychiatry and analysis of neurotics flourished.

The decade from 1952 to 1962 saw the introduction of most of the drugs that are used in psychiatry today. Reserpine, the first of the group of major tranquillisers, was soon replaced by chlorpromazine (Largactil) which was introduced in 1954. Chlordiazepoxide (Librium) heralded the minor tranquillisers in 1960, and the tricyclic antidepressants emerged to complete the three groups of drugs still most commonly prescribed.

The reduction of mental hospital population *preceded* the wide-spread introduction of drugs, reflecting a change of attitude to hospital and community treatment, a change that led to the mental health Acts of 1959 (England and Wales) and 1960 (Scotland). These Acts, in addition to providing for the safety and protection of the patient and the public, introduced two new principles: firstly, that the arrangements for the treatment of mental illness should as far as possible parallel those for the treatment of physical illness; secondly, that provision should be made for the treatment of the mentally ill in the community rather than in hospital. The most important provision was contained in a small sub-section which stated that nothing in the Act should be construed as preventing a patient who required treatment from being admitted to any hospital without any formality. In other words, as many patients as possible should be treated in the community, and those requiring hospital treatment should wherever possible be treated as voluntary patients.

The psychiatric services were becoming more aware of the need to assess and evaluate the treatment they were offering. The 'Worthing Experiment' in 1958 was the first systematic attempt to evaluate community care. Sainsbury concluded that 'a community service promotes the earlier referral of patients, thereby reducing the long period during which families suffer considerable hardship, and it can be as effective as hospital care' (Sainsbury, 1969).

Much impetus was given to the community psychiatry movement by revelations about the conditions inside some mental hospitals. Barton described *Institutional Neurosis* in 1959 and two years later Goffman, a sociologist, published *Asylums—A Study of Total Institutions*. Two other important works were published in 1961. Wing and Brown described three different mental hospitals where patients' behaviour was correlated with different hospital regimes. The same year Tooth and Brooke predicted that, if the steep decline in the hospital population continued, the large mental hospitals could be closed by the mid-70s.

The 60s proved a time of social change throughout the West, culminating in the student riots in several countries in 1968. It was also a time of therapeutic optimism. Caplan pioneered the idea of *Preventive Psychiatry* and the idea was promulgated that if only psychiatrists could become involved in everything from education to town planning, a more psychologically healthy society could be created. These wild claims for psychiatry raised expectations far in excess of what really could be delivered.

The 60s also saw the emergence of attempts to understand psychosis (e.g. Laing) and to do away with the concept of mental illness (Szasz). The Group for the Advancement of Psychiatry (G.A.P.) in 1964 declared Community Psychiatry to be the third psychiatric revolution.

The 70s brought a new realism. It was clear that the earlier estimates of the speed of decline of hospital populations were far from correct. Public enquires publicised the inhumane treatment of patients in some run-down mental hospitals. *Hospital Services for the Mentally Ill* (Department of Health and Social Security, 1971) proposed a comprehensive service based on general hospitals with an integration of community services and the gradual phasing out of the old mental hospitals in England and Wales.

The introduction of long-acting depot injections of major tranquillisers was yet another step in the right direction. This led to the setting up of continued care medication clinics and a more distinct role for community nurses. But slowly critics of the move towards community psychiatry were emerging. Hawkes (1975) asked if this was not merely another distraction from the care of the chronically ill. It also became clear that local authorities were not providing the hostels and other support services that were required. In 1983, a further GAP report, entitled *Community Care: A Reappraisal*, questioned the assumptions upon which community psychiatry was based and commented on the paucity of good research to justify these assumptions.

Twenty years or so after the last mental health legislation, further Mental Health Acts were introduced in England and Wales (1983) and Scotland (1984). The basic tenets of the previous Acts remain unchanged but with the decreased average length of treatment, the period of time between reviews of detention orders is reduced. Also, for the first time, compulsory patients are allowed the right to refuse treatment and to have a second opinion.

HISTORY—LEARNING FROM MISTAKES

This review of the development of our present way of working is necessarily selective. Some changes in development are perhaps given undue prominence, while other important events are briefly mentioned or omitted. It is a personal view which aims to highlight some issues which all those interested and involved in rehabilitation psychiatry might note and be stimulated to enquire further.

It is now difficult for us to understand how, in the name of helping the mentally ill, doctors and others came to treat so badly patients under their care. The torture and privation carried out prior to the 19th century, and even the tens of thousands of leucotomies carried out in the 1950s, are difficult to justify. The lesson that must be learned is that the impression that a particular form of treatment is effective is not enough. Each method of treatment or management must be objectively tested and assessed. It is only by evaluating our services that progress will be made and mistaken treatments avoided.

The 'ideal' service may not be ideal for a different population or culture or if tried on a different scale. The ideal small institutions developed into the impersonal destructive asylums partly as a result of size. Similarly, blind allegiance to a philosophy may result in suffering. While no-one could dispute that life in a caring family is better than life in an uncaring institution, the mass discharge of the chronically ill into a community with few provisions for their care seems to be cruelty carried out with the best of ideals but naively.

History catalogues the fluctuations in the quality of services for the mentally ill with the changes in economic and social climate. Not all of these variations were predictable. Unemployment may improve the quality of staff being recruited both in psychiatric nursing and in the choice of doctors training as psychiatrists. Recession brings cuts in spending and frequently a slipping of standards. Reduced nursing levels on wards may lead to doors being locked through lack of adequate observation of suicidal patients. Cut-backs in social work provision may lead to delays in discharge through lack of personnel to support families, or scarcity of hostel places.

Throughout history, the mental health services have suffered from the stigma associated with mental illness. Mental health does not attract political interest and politically determined policies appear to have moved towards community care in the mistaken belief that this will save money rather than for ideological reasons. Nor does the service attract much public support. Mental health charities attract three per cent of all money raised in Britain for medical charities. The wild claims made in the name of psychiatry in the 60s have proved to be counter-productive. They have tended to confirm the view that psychiatry is ineffective and therefore does not deserve more support.

Above all, psychiatry has suffered from the inability to communicate at any level. The jargon of psychiatry has all too often been unintelligible to patients, their families and the general public alike. Psychiatrists have not adequately explained their methods of working to other professionals involved with patients, and have failed to explain the needs of their patients to those responsible for financing services.

It is to be hoped that the appearance of sensible, 'normal' and realistic psychiatrists on radio and television programmes might make psychiatry and mental health appear less fearful and so not to be avoided. It rests upon all those involved in the delivery of mental health care, and perhaps particularly those involved in rehabilitation, to act as ambassadors to explain and de-mythologize psychiatry wherever they can.

REFERENCES

Barton R 1959 Institutional neurosis. Wright, Bristol
Bassuk E L, Gerson S 1978 Deinstitutionalization and mental health services. Scientific American 238: 46–53
Caplan G 1964 Principles of preventive psychiatry. Tavistock, London
DHSS 1971 Hospital services for the mentally ill. HMSO, London
Goffman E 1961 Asylums. Doubleday, New York reprinted 1970 by Penguin Books, London
Group for the Advancement of Psychiatry 1967 Education for community psychiatry, Report No. 64. Mental Health Materials Center, New York
Group for the Advancement of Psychiatry 1983 Community psychiatry: a reappraial, Report No. 113. Mental Health Materials Center, New York
Hawks D 1975 Community care: an analysis of assumptions. British Journal of Psychiatry 127: 176–85
Jones K 1960 Mental health and social policy 1845–1959. Routledge and Kegan Paul, London
Rosen G 1968 Madness in society. Routledge and Kegan Paul, London
Sainsbury P 1969 Social and community psychiatry. American Journal of Psychiatry 125: 1226–31
Scull A T 1982 Museums of madness. Penguin Books, London
Tooth G C and Brooke E M 1961 Trends in the mental hospital population. Lancet 1: 710–13

> 'The enormous disability associated with mental
> illness is to a large extent superimposed, preventable
> and treatable.'
>
> Gerald Caplan, 1961

2

The task

Ian Pullen

If any single factor was responsible for the decline in standards in the large asylums, it was the sheer size of the task set for them—the colossal number of patients requiring care. Yet what are the true dimensions of the problem? What proportion of the population is mentally ill, and of this number how many are in need of rehabilitation or long-term care?

Statistical sophistication came late to psychiatry. A hundred years ago, the increased availability of asylum beds led to an increase in the number of people being identified as mentally ill. This was interpreted mistakenly by some to mean that mental illness was increasing and led to the sort of scaremongering editorial in *The Times* quoted in the previous chapter.

PREVALENCE

Early attempts to measure psychiatric morbidity in the community presented an alarming picture. The two best known American surveys of the post-war period suggested that psychiatric symptoms were very common. The Midtown Manhattan Survey (1962) reported that 815 out of every 1000 New Yorkers had psychiatric symptoms. The Stirling County

13

Study (1963) suggested that 690 per 1000 of the population of an unidentified town (called 'Bristol' in the study) were 'genuine psychiatric cases'. Neither study used clinicians to assess the 'cases'. Later surveys, using clinical criteria, report much lower figures.

A New Haven Study reported that 'although psychiatric disorders were common, they were not ubiquitous. Over 80 per cent of subjects had no psychiatric diagnosis, either probably or definitely, including any type of personality disorder, anxiety reaction or minor depression' (Goldberg and Huxley, 1978).

Random population studies in Britain using tighter criteria for deciding 'a case' (such as a particular score on the General Health Questionnaire or Present State Examination which are both standardised research tools) have tended to produce lower results. Goldberg and Huxley (1980) estimate a one year prevalence rate of 250 per 1000 population. That is, in any year a quarter of the population can expect to suffer from psychiatric symptoms. Most of these symptoms will be mild and short-lived but others will become more chronic.

PATHWAYS TO PSYCHIATRIC CARE

So, starting with the estimate that in any one year 250 people out of every 1000 will have a psychiatric illness, Goldberg and Huxley describe the 'Pathway to Psychiatric Care' (Fig. 2.1).

the community		primary medical care		specialist psychiatric care	
population	morbidity in random community samples	total psychiatric morbidity attending G.P.	psychiatric morbidity identified by G.P.	total psychiatric patients	psychiatric in-patients only
1000 →	250 →	230 →	140 →	17 →	6 (per 1000) at risk per year.

Figure 2.1 The Pathway to psychiatric care. Adapted from Goldberg and Huxley (1980) *Mental Illness in the Community* with permission from the authors and publishers.

Two hundred and thirty will present themselves to their general practitioner who will detect only 140 as 'psychiatric cases'. The remainder, presenting mainly with physical symptoms, will be treated as though physically ill.

The general practitioner will treat most of the psychiatric problems he identifies with simple counselling, reassurance and medication (minor tranquillisers and antidepressants). He will refer 17 to the psychiatric services. Depending on the psychiatric condition, the attitude of the psychiatrist and the availability of community resources and hospital beds, approximately six per 1000 will find their way into a psychiatric bed.

These studies show that the vast majority of people suffering from psychiatric conditions never come near the psychiatric services. For those who do stray into psychiatric territory, psychiatric rehabilitation is involved, not only in the management of severe handicap, but with prevention.

PREVENTION

Prevention in psychiatry has been divided into primary, secondary and tertiary prevention (Caplan, 1964).

Primary prevention

This involves the prevention of illness. An example might be bereavement counselling. Grief is a normal, healthy reaction to loss, but occasionally it leads on to a depressive illness or other pathological condition. Counselling, available at the time of this life crisis might prevent this pathological change happening. Despite the extravagant claims of some psychiatrists in the sixties, evidence supporting the effectiveness of attempts at primary prevention in psychiatry is, as yet, slight.

Secondary prevention

This is the active treatment of an episode of illness in order to reduce symptoms to a minimum and return the patient to normality in the shortest possible time.

Tertiary prevention

This is the prevention (or minimising) of the handicap that occurs as a result of illness.

Rehabilitation focuses on secondary and tertiary prevention. To achieve this effectively, the notion of handicap must be understood.

HANDICAP

Most long-stay patients are handicapped in three basic ways (identified by Wing, 1961):
(1) they may have difficulties which *were present even before the onset of the illness*, such as a lack of social skills or low intelligence;
(2) they have disabilities which arise *as part of their illness*, such as hallucinations or apathy;
(3) they have secondary handicaps *as a result of having been ill*, and because of their own or other people's reactions to the illness.

Numbers 2 and 3 may merge to produce the picture of 'institutionalisation' which is described in Chapter 3.

ILLNESS

So far in this chapter 'illness' has not been defined. The American community surveys quoted above, show that the number of people identified as being mentally ill will depend on how illness is defined. If we accept too broad a concept, then the majority of the population will be found to be suffering from mental illness. That situation is not only of little practical use, but makes psychiatry look rather foolish.

In the 1960s, public attention was drawn to psychiatry by a group called the 'Anti-Psychiatrists' (Laing, Cooper, Basaglia, Szasz and others). It was a time of challenges to traditional authority and they sought to make psychiatry a political issue. The anti-psychiatrists, a heterogeneous group, considered psychiatry to be an enforcer of social control by which patients were made to conform. They stated that there is no such thing as schizophrenia. Not only does schizophrenia not exist, but it is a creation of psychiatrists.

Kendell pointed out that it is true that schizophrenia is a concept, but the same is equally true of other concepts such as tuberculosis or migraine. The fact that tuberculosis does not exist in a material sense does not stop people dying when their lungs have been destroyed by the tubicle bacillus (Kendell, 1975).

It is also true, as Scheff has pointed out, that part of the disability accompanying conditions such as schizophrenia is a result of the individual being labelled and treated as schizophrenic by other people. But does this invalidate schizophrenia as a concept? The only question should be: Is it a useful concept?

Much of the impetus of the anti-psychiatry movement came from its attack on the mental hospital as a place of degradation, segregation and confinement. But since the 1960s, psychiatry has undergone some changes.

In the late 1970s, the idea of 'critical psychiatry' arose. Critical psychiatrists believe that mental illnesses, whatever their correct interpretation and their political significance may be, do exist and that they do call for specialised understanding and help. They are 'critical' because they think psychiatry should examine itself to see to what extent the insights of recent sociology and philosophy can offer benefits to society (Ingleby, 1981).

In view of these criticisms, it is necessary to justify the use of diagnosis and the classification of psychiatric disorders. Kendell pointed out that there are three aspects to every human being: (1) those shared with all mankind; (2) those shared with some others, but not all; (3) those which are unique to him. The value of classification depends on the size of the second relative to the other two.

SCHIZOPHRENIA—THE CONCEPT

As much of the work of rehabilitation is concerned with schizophrenia, it is perhaps useful to consider the development of the concept of schizophrenia as an example of the evolution of diagnoses.

The term schizophrenia (or rather the schizophrenias) was coined by Bleuler in 1911 and was a refinement of the work published 15 years earlier by Kraepelin.

In 1896, Kraepelin divided the functional psychoses (then considered to be the type of insanity not caused by physical or organic disease) into two groups: those that always recovered, however long the recovery might be delayed; and those where recovery was never complete (Fig. 2.2). This latter group he called dementia praecox. This was diagnosis by prognosis (outcome), the two groups being distinguished by whether or not they recovered completely.

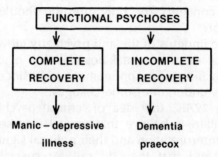

Figure 2.2 Kraepelin's classification, i.e. diagnosis by prognosis

Bleuler widened the concept of dementia praecox by adding a group of patients who showed a similar deterioration but without ever becoming overtly psychotic (hallucinated or deluded). These patients, now called schizophrenics, all shared four fundamental symptoms: (1) loosening of association (no coherent train of thought); (2) autism (failure of social communication); (3) ambivalence; (4) disturbances of mood (blunting/incongruity). This was diagnosis by symptomatology. Unfortunately, these four symptoms are impossible to define and all-embracing, and so attempts have been made to specify precisely which symptoms to use. One example is Schneider's Symptoms of the First Rank.

First rank symptoms of schizophrenia are:

— thought insertion (experience of thoughts being put into one's mind);

— thought withdrawal (experience of thoughts being taken out of one's mind);
— thought broadcasting (experience of one's thoughts being known to others);
— feelings of passivity (experience of emotions, specific bodily movements or specific sensations being caused by a external agency or being under some external control);
— voices discussing one's thoughts or behaviour, as they occur, sometimes forming a running commentary;
— voices discussing or arguing about one, referring to 'he';
— voices repeating one's thoughts out loud or anticipating one's thoughts;
— primary delusions, arising inexplicably from perceptions which in themselves are normal (for example, 'I know that I am God because the traffic lights changed to green,').

Although Schneider's symptoms correspond fairly well to the existing concept of schizophrenia in Britain, they were not the result of research and only about 70 per cent of patients diagnosed in Britain as suffering from schizophrenia will have first rank symptoms. The International Classification of Diseases produced by the World Health Organization spells out in more detail the group of symptoms that justify the diagnosis of schizophrenia.

Few contemporary psychiatrists are entirely happy with our present classification, because of the diversity of presentation, features and prognoses under each diagnostic category. Even fewer would regard either manic depressive illness or schizophrenia as disease entities but rather as clusters of symptoms. We continue to use this system, if only because it is familiar and we have nothing better to put in its place (Kendell, 1975).

DIAGNOSIS

It may be helpful at this stage to think about the need for diagnosis, especially as the diagnostic categories may not represent disease entities *per se*, and they may be applied in a fashion that brings their reliability into question. But all those working within rehabilitation should be able to understand and justify the system that they use.

Disadvantages

The disadvantages of diagnosis are:
(1) *False sense of security.* We may quickly forget that it was quite difficult to assign the patient to a particular diagnosis, so that 'a possible case of schizophrenia' may soon be referred to as 'this schizophrenic'.
(2) *Labelling.* Once a diagnostic label is applied, it alters the patient's expectations, as well as those of his relatives, employer and not least the clinical team.
(3) *Inadequacy.* Every person is unique and the diagnosis is pitifully inadequate when faced with conveying the complexity of a person's predicament.
(4) *Pejorative.* Some diagnoses imply value judgements, such as 'personality disorder'.

Menninger (1963) called for the abandonment of diagnosis and 'using no names at all for the conditions of mental illness'. Instead there should be a lengthy formulation of each person's predicament.

These dangers and shortcomings of diagnosis must be balanced against the advantages, if a diagnosis is to be made.

Advantages

The advantages of diagnosis are:
(1) *Predictive.* It will give some indication of the natural history of the condition so that a prognosis can be given. It will predict which treatment is likely to be beneficial and, equally important, where no treatment will be helpful or should be offered.
(2) *Confidence.* Even a 'bad' diagnosis gives the patient and relatives a feeling of relief that there is an explanation for what has been happening, that this condition is shared with other people. They are not alone and unique and the staff know what is wrong.
(3) *Research, progress and planning.* Research depends on identifying groups of people with the same condition to be allocated to different methods of treatment or management. Without diagnostic groups, no logical progress can be made. Similarly, epidemiological research depends on studying different groups of diagnoses to establish common aetiologi-

cal factors in the hope of prevention and for planning the services they will require.

(4) *Communication*. A diagnosis is a short-hand way of communicating quite complex information about an individual.

So, despite all the shortcomings and reservations, for the foreseeable future, classification of diagnoses is inescapable. Without it, no progress can be made, no treatment logically given, nor realistic expectations and rehabilitation plans made.

CLASSIFICATION

As this book is intended for all members of the multidisciplinary team, it is worth reviewing the classification in some detail to ensure that, when diagnosis is used in discussion, all members of the team are talking about the same concept. It was a salutary lesson to learn that there are not many more schizophrenics in the USA than in Britain, but that American psychiatrists mean something different when they use the term. The US/UK Diagnostic Project clearly demonstrated, using standard diagnostic criteria (Present State Examination), that the same patient might receive a different label, not only on opposite sides of the Atlantic, but also across the States. There is much room for confusion and, wherever possible, this must be avoided. A glossary such as ICD-9 (WHO, 1978) is useful.

Some definitions

Neurosis

The patient usually retains insight and has unimpaired reality testing; that is he knows that his experiences are part of an illness, even though he is unable to do anything about them. The symptoms are only *quantitatively* different from normality in that the symptoms differ from normal experience only in degree. Thus someone suffering from an anxiety neurosis will have symptoms indistinguishable from normal anxiety, the sort of feelings anyone would experience in an anxiety-provoking situation such as a job interview or examination.

However these symptoms occur out of context or are more prolonged or severe than the situation warrants. Empathy is not difficult.

Neurosis: insight
     in touch with reality
     quantitatively different
     empathy possible.

Examples of neuroses: anxiety neurosis
     depressive neurosis
     obsessional neurosis
     phobic neurosis
     hysterical neurosis

Psychosis

In general, patients suffering from psychosis do not recognise that they are ill or that their experiences (hallucinations, delusions) are part of illness. That is, they have no insight and have lost touch with reality. The experiences are *qualitatively* different from normal experience. Hopefully, we will not have hallucinations or become unshakeably convinced that we are being attacked by X-rays, and it is difficult for us to appreciate just what it must be like to have these experiences.

Psychosis: lack of insight
     out of touch with reality
     qualitatively different
     empathy difficult

Examples of psychosis: schizophrenia
     manic depressive psychosis
     organic states (dementia, acute confusion)

The distinction between neurosis and psychosis is difficult and remains subject to debate. Neuroses and psychoses are illnesses: they have a beginning then run their course, but, most important of all, there was a time before which the illness was not present (Fig. 2.3). Illness is therefore superimposed on whatever personality the individual has.

Personality is that unique combination of qualities that distinguishes each of us from our fellows. This includes our

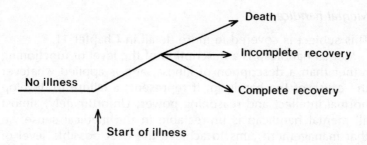

Figure 2.3 The course of an illness.

predominant mood, how we react to stress, the sort of relationships we make, our moral values, our sensitiveness, stability of mood, personal security and so on, and from our early 20s these features remain relatively stable. So the way we react to certain circumstances now will be very similar to the way we will respond in five or ten years time.

Personality disorder

Personality is said to be disordered when it differs significantly from what is accepted as 'normal', either in the balance of its components, their quality and expression or in its total aspect. If this definition appears unduly vague and therefore of little use, that is precisely what it is. This diagnosis depends on a mixture of objective evidence from the case history such as patterns of relationships and behaviour, plus a subjective response of the psychiatrist to the individual at interview. It is, therefore, a most unreliable diagnostic entity and should seldom be used. The label of personality disorder carries pejorative connotations often involving value judgements. As there is little evidence that anything other than time alters personality, a diagnosis of personality disorder often appears a way of depriving someone of help.

Examples of personality disorder: paranoid
schizoid
explosive
obsessional
inadequate
antisocial

Mental handicap

This subject is covered in more detail in Chapter 11.

Mental handicap is a description of the level of functioning rather than a description of illness, and is applied whatever the cause of the handicap. It represents a failure to develop normal intellect and reasoning power. Unfortunately, almost all mental handicap is untreatable in the medical sense, so that management aims to achieve the best possible level of functioning for each individual depending on his degree of handicap.

THE RELIABILITY OF DIAGNOSIS

Some diagnostic categories appear considerably more reliable than others. Kreitman and his colleagues in Chichester set out to study the reliability of diagnoses made by six pairs of psychiatrists. The study was important in that interviews were held in ordinary NHS working conditions. The consultants obtained 75 per cent agreement for organic diagnoses (e.g. dementia) and 61 per cent for functional psychoses (manic depressive illness and schizophrenia), but only 28 per cent agreement for neurotic disorders. In other words reliability, particularly for non-psychotic conditions, is low (Kreitman, 1961).

The reliability in research situations has been improved by the use of standardised research tools such as the Present State Examination, with which levels of agreement for diagnoses such as schizophrenia can rise above 90 per cent (Wing et al, 1974).

THE OUTCOME OF ILLNESS

Many aetiological factors are thought to be involved in the production of psychiatric illness and in its maintenance once it is established. Although for many conditions these factors are imperfectly understood, it appears that the functional psychoses (schizophrenia and manic depressive illness) have a genetic (inherited) component, approximately 10–15 per cent of first degree relatives manifesting a similar illness. Other aetiological factors include psychological and physical stresses, physical illness and other insults such as drug and alcohol abuse and withdrawal.

The eventual outcome of any illness will depend upon the nature of the condition, the extent to which precipitating factors such as family stresses can be relieved, the benefits for the patient of retaining the 'sick role', and to what extent the process can be modified by treatment. Different diagnostic groups carry different natural histories. For example, the neuroses tend to improve spontaneously over time, two-thirds having recovered or considerably improved within two years. On the other hand, some neuroses will continue to plague patients for the rest of their lives. Some conditions, such as manic depressive illness, may produce cycles of illness and complete recovery, while schizophrenia tends to recover incompletely.

This variety of outcomes was well-known to the ancient Greeks who described the possibilites outlined in Figure 2.3.

PROBLEMS OF RECURRENT ILLNESS

Partial, or even complete recovery from an episode of psychiatric illness brings in its wake a number of stresses related to coming to terms with the idea of having been ill, coping with other people's changed attitudes to the 'ex-patient' and facing the uncertainty of whether and when the condition might return. With recurrent illness, it is this latter factor which assumes greatest importance.

Employers might tolerate one spell of illness sympathetically, but begin to consider retirement 'on health grounds' if the illness returns. Planning at work or for the family at home becomes difficult when a person is faced with uncertainty in the future. The stress will also be felt by those most closely involved emotionally, and this may completely alter a marital relationship.

For all these reasons, it is vital to start treatment as soon as possible in a new episode of illness, and to consider the merits of keeping the patient away from work to avoid poor performance or disturbance that might make return to work more difficult. Those closest to the patient should be involved in treatment and offered practical help and support.

THE NEW CHRONICS

A generation of psychiatric patients has now been exposed to 'community care' of which an important concept is avoidance, wherever possible, of long-term in-patient care. The decline in the number of non-geriatric long-term beds has meant that many patients who would previously have been resident in hospital are out in the community. However, much psychiatric illness runs a chronic course and inevitably some patients still need to remain in hospital for long periods of time (Macreadie, 1983).

The 'new chronics' are defined as patients aged 18–64 who have been in hospital for more than one but less than six years. Recent surveys in England and Wales (1976) and Scotland (1983) show the bed occupancy for 'new chronics' to be about 20 per 100 000 of the general population. Although for the whole group schizophrenia was the most common diagnosis, the majority of first admissions had a diagnosis of organic brain disease (pre-senile dementia and alcoholic psychosis) even though this is for the pre-geriatric age group.

Those patients who, during their first hospital admission, stay long enough to be a 'new chronic', are usually found to be so disabled as to be considered well placed in hospital (5.8 beds per 100 000 population). The reasons for remaining in hospital are not always medical. Of the new chronics surveyed, it was thought that 38 per cent did not need in-patient care and could have been discharged if other supported places had been available, and 20 per cent could have been accommodated in staffed hostels.

GRADUATE PATIENTS

We live in an ageing population. The reasons for this are covered in more detail in Chapter 12. Many patients who came into hospital as young people are now growing old within the system. When they reach the age of 65, they may be called 'graduates'.

As a group, graduates tend to be treated separately from psychogeriatric patients, many of whom will be suffering from dementia. However, increased age brings increased frailty and the probability of physical illness. Staffing levels and expectations will have to alter to match the needs of this particular group.

CONCLUSIONS: CLASSIFICATION OR CONFUSION?

Although almost a quarter of the population will experience psychiatric symptoms in any given year, very few develop serious psychiatric illnesses. Despite the shortcomings of the present classification, it is necessary to arrive at a diagnosis before any logical treatment or management plans can be made. Schizophrenia, the most common diagnosis in rehabilitation work, is one of the more reliable diagnostic entities. The lesson is that a diagnosis, once made, is not applied for life but should be reviewed critically from time to time.

REFERENCES

Caplan G 1961 An approach to community mental health. Tavistock, London
Caplan G 1964 Principles of preventive psychiatry. Tavistock, London
Cooper J E, Kendell R E, Gurland B J, Sharpe L, Copeland J R M, Simon R 1972 Psychiatric diagnosis in New York and London. Maudsley Monograph No. 20. Oxford University Press, London
Goldberg D, Huxley P 1980 Mental illness in the community: The pathway to psychiatric care. Tavistock, London
Ingleby D 1981 Critical psychiatry: the politics of mental health. Penguin, London
Kendell R E 1975 The role of diagnosis in psychiatry. Blackwell, Oxford
Kreitman N 1961 The reliability of psychiatric diagnosis. Journal of Mental Science 107: 876–86
Leighton D C, Harding J C, Macklin D M, Macmillan A M, Leighton A H 1963 The character of danger [Stirling County]. Basic Books, New York
Macreadie R G, Oliver A, Wilson A, Burton L L 1983 The Scottish survey of 'new chronic' inpatients. British Journal of Psychiatry 143: 564–71
Mann S A, Cree W 1976 'New' long-stay psychiatric inpatients: a national sample survey of fifteen mental hospitals in England and Wales 1972/3. Psychological Medicine 6: 603–16

Menninger K 1963 The Vital Balance. Viking Press, New York

Schneider K 1959 Clinical psychopathology. Grune and Stratton, New York

Stole L, Langer T, Michael S, Opiler M, Rennie T 1962 Mental health in the metropolis [Manhattan]. McGraw-Hill, New York

WHO 1978 Mental disorders: glossary and guide to their classification in accordance with the ninth revision of the international classification of diseases. World Health Organization, Geneva

Wing J K 1963 Rehabilitation of psychiatric patients. British Journal of Psychiatry 109: 635–41

Wing J K, Cooper J E, Sartorius N 1974 Description and classification of psychiatric symptoms. Cambridge University Press, Cambridge

Home is home, though it be never so homely.

John Clare, 1630

3

Where?

Ian Pullen

The shift from hospital to community care which began in the mid-1950s brought about a questioning of the long-term effects of hospital stay on the patient. In the 1960s Goffman and Barton spelt out, more explicitly, the undesirable effects of institutions.

HOME VERSUS HOSPITAL

In 1964, community psychiatry was proclaimed the third psychiatric revolution. (The first two being Pinel's unchaining of the insane and Freud's discovery of psychoanalysis.) The concept of community psychiatry involved psychiatrists accepting responsibility for a catchment population, promoting mental health, prevention, earlier involvement with patients and earlier treatment and, above all, the idea of treating people wherever possible in their own surroundings and keeping the length of time spent in hospital to a minimum.

There were strong advocates of the new system and in 1967, the American Group for the Advancement of Psychiatry enthusiastically supported 'this emerging sub-specialty of psychiatry'. But not everyone shared this enthusiasm. Kubie, in America, feared that community psychiatry would 'suffer the fate of all good intentions not guided by mature judgement and experience'. Dunham called it 'the newest therapeutic bandwagon' while in Britain, Hawks considered it another distraction from the care of the chronically ill (Hawks, 1975), and feared that it would attract resources and interest away from psychiatry's main task of treating and caring for those with genuine mental illness.

In other words, the critics feared that the untested ideals of community care would not lead to better community mental health but instead divert resources away from the treatment of those who were chronically ill.

THEORY OF COMMUNITY PSYCHIATRY

The Group for the Advancement of Psychiatry summarised community psychiatry as 'the application and practice of psychiatry in non-institutional and relatively non-traditional settings'. It has the following characteristics:

— It is based on the assumption that socio-cultural conditions significantly influence the manifestations and course of psychiatric illness.
— It studies the role of social environment in psychiatric illness.
— It is concerned with the organisation and delivery of mental health services.
— It uses social and environmental measures to prevent psychiatric illness and to treat and care for those who develop psychiatric disorders.
— It supplies treatment and care as close as possible to the patient's home or work place.
— It uses community resources to extend services beyond the more conventional psychiatric treatment settings.

In short, it sets out to provide care for the psychiatrically ill as close to their homes as possible and to direct efforts towards prevention of psychiatric illness.

The decision to admit

In the past, the decision to admit a patient to hospital was a more or less automatic response to certain diagnoses. So, a diagnosis of schizophrenia or psychosis with the presence of hallucinations and delusions meant certain admission. In some British hospitals, within the past 20 years, the family doctor, whose knowledge of psychiatry might be slight, had the right to admit patients direct to the wards.

Well, what is wrong with this? As we shall see later, the decision to admit should *not* be taken lightly as it carries serious implications for the patient's future.

The presence of hallucinations will have a very different significance depending on whether they started last week or have been present for years. In general, it is not the number or even the severity of symptoms that is important, but rather how much of the healthy person remains. So we need to consider how the person is functioning *in spite of the symptoms* and also what stresses and supports are present if we are to make a sensible decision about how and where best to provide treatment.

Debilitating effects of institutions

The problems are of two kinds: (1) long-stay institutions appear to lead to the development of an 'institutional syndrome' which makes the patient less fit for life outside the institution; (2) mere admission to mental hospital stigmatises the patient. The attitudes and expectations of the patient, as well as those of people about him, change as a result of being in hospital. This affects the chances of successful adjustment back into the community.

THE 'INSTITUTIONAL SYNDROME'

Barton (1959) and Goffman (1961) described the institutional syndrome which is characterised by:
— apathy
— lack of initiative
— loss of interest (in things or events not immediately personal or present)
— submissiveness
— lack of expression of feeling or resentment of harsh or unfair orders from staff

— loss of individuality
— deterioration in personal habits, toilet and general standards.

There is a resigned acceptance that things will go on as they are 'unchangingly, inevitably and indefinitely'.

How does this state of acceptance, passivity and apathy arise? It appears to be a result of at least three factors including the disease process itself, a restricted life-style prior to admission, and the effects of institutional life. Hospital admission not only separates the patient from the world outside, but also takes over virtually all decision-making and functions for self-preservation. Wing (1961), studying a group of patients who had spent more than two years in hospital, found that the longer the stay in hospital, the more unfavourable the patient's attitude to discharge.

Barton suggested eight aetiological factors associated with the institutional syndrome:
(1) loss of contact with the outside world
(2) enforced idleness
(3) brutality, brow-beating and teasing
(4) bossiness of the staff
(5) loss of personal friends, possessions and personal events (e.g. birthdays)
(6) drugs
(7) ward atmosphere
(8) loss of prospects outside the institution.

If Barton's suggestions are correct, and remember that they have not been specifically tested, then it would suggest that the institutional syndrome should be reduced by altering these factors, or should be less likely to occur if patients are treated in the community. Presumably, the more the patient is in touch with the community, the less likely he is to lose contact with the 'real' world, personal friends, possessions and personal events. The prevailing ward atmosphere, domineering or even cruel ward staff, should of course be looked for and where possible changed.

But changing systems is not as simple as might at first appear. Firstly, people in institutions tend to resist change and, even when identified, undesirable attitudes might prove very difficult to change. Secondly, even where there is a desire to change, the precise changes brought about might not be what one had anticipated.

A recent study in a Scottish psychiatric hospital monitored staff and patient activity in a psychogeriatric ward during several thousand 30-second time intervals. The first measurements were taken in an old ward of poor design with toilets and dining room situated at a distance from the sitting room. Over 60% of the patients' time was spent in total inactivity. Thirty per cent of their time was devoted to self-care (dressing, toileting) and eating. The measurements were repeated after a move to a purpose-built psychogeriatric unit of compact design and with increased nursing levels. Time spent in total inactivity increased to 75% and self-care reduced to 15%. Although 10% of the time was spent in staff-patient contact (including medical staff and occupational therapist) the time nurses spent in contact with patients, except where they were giving instructions, dispensing medication or applying dressings, was only 1½% of the patients' day. Thus, nurses were spending only 20 seconds per hour talking to an individual patient. The compact design of the ward meant that nurses spent less time taking patients to and from the toilet and meals. The increased nursing levels paradoxically reduced their contact with patients and increased the nurse to nurse interaction. For example, in under-staffed wards where one nurse would help a patient dress, the nurse talked to the patient. If two nurses dressed a patient, the nurses tended to talk to each other.

But it is not only prolonged spells in hospital that produce problems. *Any* hospital admission may have adverse effects. These adverse effects include:
— Crisis of admission (the stress of going into hospital)
— Stigma
— Changes of attitude, lowered expectations
— Increased risk of readmission
— Poorer social adjustment, financial costs to the family
— Crisis of discharge.

For many people, admission to a psychiatric hospital or psychiatric ward in a general hospital is a terrifying experience. This results partly from ignorance and fantasies about 'madness'. But part of the fear is based in reality. The revolving door policy propels patients out of hospital at an earlier stage in their recovery so that as soon as people show signs of improvement, they are discharged. Also, alternatives such as acute day hospitals, now cope with many patients who only a few years ago would have been treated in hospital. Wards tend to contain a concentration of bizarre and disturbed behaviour that, a few years ago, would have been diluted with a larger number of recovered or recovering patients. Thus, many psychiatric wards are disturbed and disturbing.

Hospital admission affects the attitude and expectations of the patient, his family and other important people such as his employer. Doctors are not immune to this influence. Mendel and Rapport showed that a history of previous admissions greatly influenced the doctor towards a decision to readmit the patient. So the decision to admit a patient for the first time may affect the rest of his life. Under stress, the patient's expectations may well be that he will not cope, and in the event of being seen by a psychiatrist, he is more likely to end up in hospital again.

Attempts to combat the institutional syndrome

What can be done to modify the effect of the institution on a patient? Barton suggested the following:

(1) re-establishment of patient's contacts—with ward, hospital functions, patient's home and catchment area,

(2) provision of a daily sequence of useful occupations, recreations and social events 14 hours a day, seven days a week: ward programmes, shaving, grooming, toilet, dressing and self-care; redevelopment of social skills and graces; cooking and household management; recreation; physical exercise; work;

(3) eradication of brutality, brow-beating and teasing;

(4) alteration of the attitude of professional staff;

(5) encouragement (and possibility) for a patient to have friends, possessions and to enjoy personal events;

(6) reduction of drugs;

(7) provision of a homely, friendly, permissive ward atmosphere;

(8) making the patient aware of prospects of accommodation, work and friends outside hospital.

How do Barton's suggestions stand up to scrutiny 20 years after they were first proposed? Undoubtedly, the attitude of professional staff and their contact with patients must at all times be monitored and attempts made, where necessary, to modify the way they relate to patients in their care. Provision must be made for patients to spend more time out of the ward and hospital and among normal people. Links must be maintained with friends and family, encouraging them not only to visit the patient in hospital but also to take him out to his familiar surroundings. For many chronically ill patients, the ward will remain their home for many months or years. They have a right to live in a homely atmosphere with adequate privacy and to be surrounded by personal possessions.

Perhaps the two suggestions which, in the light of current experience, we might disagree with are numbers (2) and (6). The idea of anyone (ourselves included!) devoting 14 hours a day, seven days a week to 'useful occupations, recreations and social events' is daunting. There is a danger that any attempt to provide this amount of stimulation and structure would lead to the provision of large group activities and the re-creation of institutional behaviour. While, at first glance, the idea of every patient joining in for a keep-fit routine first thing in the morning might seem healthy, dealing with a group *en masse* reduces staff-patient interaction and allows the patient to 'switch off'. Less activity, but tailored to the needs of the individual, is more appropriate. The reduction of drugs, usually major tranquillisers, is only appropriate where over-prescribing is the practice. Many patients may be less able to take part in rehabilitation activities if they are under-medicated (see chapter on treatment).

Research evidence

Stein and Test (1978) draw attention to the research evaluating the effect of more humane, pleasant hospital environments. While such treatment does appear to be correlated with adjustment in hospital, it is unrelated to discharge rates or post-hospital adjustment. Wing and Brown (1961) surveyed three mental hospitals identified by the letters A, B and C. The subjects were female patients under the age of sixty, with a diagnosis of schizophrenia, who had spent more than two years in hospital. The patient's mental state, behaviour in the ward and attitude to discharge were assessed, as was the ward (ward restrictiveness scores). A consistent pattern emerged. At Hospital A, where the main emphasis of care was on the long-stay patients, there was least clinical disturbance and most personal freedom, useful occupation, and optimism among the nursing staff. At Hospital C, where progress had been slower, there was most clinical disturbance among patients and least personal freedom, useful occupation and optimism. Hospital B was intermediate.

This was good preliminary evidence that social conditions in mental hospitals do influence the mental state of schizophrenic patients. The longer-term study (Wing and Brown, 1970) concluded that a substantial proportion, though by no means all, of the morbidity shown by long-stay schizophrenic patients in mental hospitals is a product of their environment.

Poverty of social environment (fewest personal possessions, little contact with the world outside and pessimistic nurses) was very highly correlated with a clinical poverty syndrome (institutionalism). It appeared that schizophrenic patients may be vulnerable to under-stimulating environments wherever they occur, in hospital or in the community.

That the rehabilitation process precipitated relapse of florid symptoms could not be ruled out by the studies and should be borne in mind.

Clearly the most important single factor associated with clinical improvement (primary handicap) was a reduction in the amount of time doing nothing. The only important category distinguishing patients who improved clinically from those who did not was work and occupational therapy.

This work has been quoted extensively because of its great importance for the field of rehabilitation. It is the only systematic study of different hospitals and different social environments over a period of years, and it has answered many basic questions.

Linn (1970) went further by looking at a wider range of variables, and found that discharge rates were unrelated to 'humane treatment' (hospital atmosphere, good facilities, humanistic policies). These findings are similar to those for other types of in-patient treatment such as therapeutic communities and token economy wards, both of which have been shown to improve behaviour and change attitudes within the institution, but this progress is not maintained after discharge.

These negative findings should not detract from the very real need to improve standards of care and humanity within institutions. If there are doubts about the effects that institutions have on patients, then what of attempts to reduce the amount of time spent in hospital?

ATTEMPTS TO REDUCE THE LENGTH OF HOSPITAL STAY

In 1978, researchers in Edinburgh and London were tackling this problem. Noting the trend towards shorter hospital admissions in British mental hospitals, both teams set out to assess the effects of very short stays in hospital. They randomly allocated patients to a 'short stay' or 'normal stay' ward. The 'short stay' patients spent less than half the length of time in hospital compared with the normal patients (Kennedy, Hirsch). It appears that patients often get better in time for discharge.

In the United States, Caffey et al (1968) randomly allocated newly admitted schizophrenic patients to one of three treatments: (1) normal hospital care with usual after-care; (2) brief intensive treatment with special after-case; and (3) normal hospital care with special after-care. The brief treatment lasted an average of 29 days compared with 83 for the other two forms, but the readmission rates were not significantly different and overall the 'brief group' spent less time in hospital.

In summary, these studies show that brief hospital admission is as effective as longer admission. Although these patients spend less time in hospital, the total amount of time spent in contact with the hospital (for example, as day patients) may be longer. Although the relapse rate is identical to that of the longer stay patients, it has been shown that as hospital admissions get shorter, in some cases readmission rates increase.

ATTEMPTS TO TREAT WITHOUT HOSPITAL ADMISSION

A further step in the attempt to avoid the debilitating effects of hospital admission is to try to avoid hospital admission altogether. In Denver, Langsley studied a group of patients for whom it had been decided that hospital admission was necessary. Providing they lived within one hour's travelling time from the hospital, lived with their family and were not homicidal, they were randomly allocated to normal hospital admission or sent home to be treated by the Family Crisis Therapy Team (FCT). The FCT group of patients were In touch with the crisis team for an average of 24 days. The control group who were admitted to hospital as usual spent an average of 29 days in hospital (Table 3.1).

Table 3.1 Family Crisis Therapy (Langsley, Machotka and Flomenhaft, 1971).

Family crisis therapy (FCT)	Normal hospital admission (control group)
24.2 *days* average contact 4.2 clinic visits 1.3 home visits 5.4 telephone calls 1.2 contacts with other agencies	28.6 *days* average in hospital

During the study period, none of the patients allocated to FCT needed to be admitted. (Remember, all of these patients had been thought to require hospital admission at the time they entered the study.) During the six months after the study, fewer of the FCT patients required readmission (13% compared with 29% of those that had been in hospital).

Although patients treated at home got better at the same rate as those in hospital—no faster but no slower—on social adjustment scores, those treated at home seemed to have fewer problems as a result of the illness. Finally, it was calculated that treatment at home cost one sixth of that of hospital treatment.

This work has been replicated by Fenton in Montreal with similar conclusions. So it appears that a wide range of mentally ill patients can be treated as effectively at home as they are in hospital providing they have a supportive family. But many of our patients have lost contact with their families, have no surviving family or, as is often the case, have no family who are *prepared* to look after them. For this group, we have to fall back on day hospital, group homes, hostels (half-way houses) and supported flats and lodgings.

Day versus in-patient care

Day hospitals have been used both as a transition between in-patient care and the community, and as an alternative to 24 hour care. Although descriptive studies of day hospital treatment are enthusiastic, 'Controlled studies comparing the effectiveness of day versus in-patient treatment are scarce' (Stein and Test, 1978). One study (Herz et al, 1971) randomly allocated patients to either day or in-patient treatment. They reported that the day patients spent significantly less time in contact with the hospital, had a lower readmission rate than in-patients, and scored lower on several measures of symptomatology. However, such research has several limitations. The studies performed so far have excluded from day hospitals a large number of patients regarded as too disturbed and readmission rates following day hospital treatment remain high.

Half-way houses

Half-way houses or hospital hostels are another possibility for the treatment of the chronically disturbed or impaired patient. These facilities, with an emphasis on re-socialisation and re-settlement, have been used mainly as a transition from hospital to the community.

Controlled research on half-way houses and hostels is almost entirely lacking, but again descriptive reports are encouraging. A major problem is again a high hospital readmission rate, in part due to the fact that many patients have a recurrence of severe symptoms when pushed to 'move on' to a more independent life after leaving the half-way house (Stein and Test, 1978).

ATTEMPTS TO TREAT CHRONIC PATIENTS IN THE COMMUNITY

Marx et al (1973) decided to try community treatment for a group of patients still in hospital and who were not considered to be capable of 'sustained community living'. The patients were randomly allocated to an experimental group and a control group. The experimental group of patients spent up to eight days in the research ward for assessment before being sent out into the community regardless of their symptoms. The control patients either stayed on their wards or were sent to a research ward for five months training before being discharged.

As chronic patients are prone to drop out of treatment if they have to attend a clinic, the experimental treatment involved staff going out to the patients. Staff spent much of the day and evening alongside the patients, teaching coping skills and helping them to acquire skills of daily living such as cooking and self-care. This treatment lasted for five months after which the patients were linked in with the usual community services. These unselected chronically symptomatic patients managed well in the community. Only one out of 21 experimental patients required hospital admission during the five month period, and then only for one day. During the two years of follow-up, this group gained a significantly higher level of independent living than the control group, although over a time, the difference between the two groups diminished.

Criticisms of the experiments

A great deal of time and effort has gone into all the experimental evaluations described above. Undoubtedly they tell us more about what might be achieved but caution must be exercised when trying to apply these results to 'real' services.

The short-stay experiments described by Kennedy and Hirsch ran for only about one year and the FCT services described by Langsley and Fenton only lasted for a limited period. The enthusiasm required for this sort of work, together with the considerable stresses involved in managing difficult patients outside hospital, may be tolerated for the period of an experiment, especially where the experimenters have a vested interest in demonstrating that the new service can work. What the experiments have demonstrated is that patients can be managed in this particular way, certainly for a limited period of time. We require longer term evaluation of 'real' services running over several years before we can be sure of the longer term effects on patients, their families and staff. At present, we should remain guardedly optimistic.

Does it save money?

It was thought that closing expensive mental hospitals and caring for patients in the community would be cheaper, and hence the idea was very popular with politicians. Langsley calculated that FCT treatment for his patients cost only one sixth of that of hospital admission. Weisprod, Test and Stein carried out an extensive cost/benefit analysis of their community care service in Wisconsin and found that patient care in either hospital or community setting was very high. The hospital-based programme was about 10 per cent cheaper per patient, but taking all benefits and costs into account, the community programme provided some benefits to patients not supplied by the hospital service.

Further research is required to answer this question. But to provide as high a standard of care to patients in the community as is offered to those in hospital may not produce the massive savings that had been anticipated. This must be weighed against the benefits, for the patient, in terms of independence and normality of life possible in the community.

There is a grave danger of recreating institutions in the community. Life in an inadequately supervised and unstimulating lodging house may reproduce all the faults of the old mental hospital. We must ensure that community care does not turn into community carelessness.

REFERENCES

Barton R 1959 Institutional neurosis. Wright, Bristol

Caffey E M, Jones R B, Diamond L S, et al 1968 Brief hospital treatment of schizophrenia: early results of a multiple hospital study. Hospital and Community Psychiatry 19: 282–7

Dunham H W 1965 Community psychiatry, the newest therapeutic bandwagon. Archives of General Psychiatry 12: 303–13

Fenton F R, Tessier L, Struening E L, Smith F A, Benoit C 1982 Home and hospital psychiatric treatment. Croom Helm, London

Goffman E 1961 Asylums. Doubleday, New York reprinted 1970 by Penguin Books, London

Group for the Advancement of Psychiatry 1967 Education for community psychiatry, Report No. 64. Mental Health Materials Center, New York

Group for the Advancement of Psychiatry 1983 Community psychiatry: a reappraisal, Report No. 113. Mental Health Materials Center, New York

Hawks D 1975 Community care: an analysis of assumptions. British Journal of Psychiatry 127: 176–85

Hirsch S R, Platt S, Knights A, Weyman A 1979 Shortening hospital stay for psychiatric care: effect on patients and their families. British Medical Journal 1: 442–6

Kennedy P, Hird F 1980 Description and evaluation of a short-stay admission ward. British Journal of Psychiatry 136: 205–15

Kubie L 1968 Pitfalls of community psychiatry. Archives of General Psychiatry 18: 257–66

Langsley D G, Machotka P, Flomenhaft M S W 1971 Avoiding mental hospital admission: a follow-up study. American Journal of Psychiatry 127: 1391–4

Linn L S 1970 State hospital environments and rates of patient discharge. Archives of General Psychiatry 23: 346–51

Marx A J, Test M A, Stein L I 1973 Extrohospital management of severe mental illness. Archives of General Psychiatry 29: 205–11

Mendel W M, Rapport S 1978 Determinants of the decision for psychiatric hospitalisation. Archives of General Psychiatry 20: 321–8

Stein L I, Test M A 1978 Alternatives to mental hospital treatment. Plenum Press, New York

Stein L I, Test M A 1980 Alternative to mental hospital treatment. Archives of General Psychiatry 37: 392–7

Wing J K 1961 A simple and reliable subclassification of chronic schizophrenia. Journal of Mental Science 107: 862–75

Wing J K, Brown G W 1961 Social treatment of schizophrenia: a comparative survey of three mental hospitals. Journal of Mental Science 107: 847–61

Wing J K, Brown G W 1970 Institutionalism and schizophrenia: a comparative study of three mental hospitals 1960–1968. Cambridge University Press, London

Any patient, however seemingly intractable the condition, retains the capacity to surprise the persistent therapist.

Wing and Brown, 1971

4

Principles of rehabilitation

Clephane Hume

WHAT IS REHABILITATION?

Rehabilitation is the process through which a person is helped to adjust to the limitations of his disability. Lost skills may be regained and coping strategies developed. The nature of the impairment dictates the particular focus of rehabilitation, but at all times the patient must be treated as an individual. The complexity and variety of problems presented must never be allowed to obscure the individual's needs. Ultimately, the focus of rehabilitation must be the quality of a patient's life.

The rehabilitation process cannot be undertaken in isolation: family and friends, fellow patients and staff all play a part. Nor can the process be carried out in a hospital vacuum: the realities of the outside world must be considered and treatment extended into the community prior to resettlement.

Rehabilitation means systematic work for patients and staff over long periods of time. Though achievements may be reached only slowly and even painfully, the results can be rewarding.

AIMS OF REHABILITATION

The aim of rehabilitation is to restore the individual to his

43

maximum level of independence, psychologically, socially, physically and economically.

In this definition 'maximum level' means the optimum level for that individual and therefore it is inappropriate to define a general standard. This means that success is an individual matter to be judged in terms of the goals set for that person. For many, discharge will be a realistic aim, but for others a more independent level of living within hospital may be the appropriate goal.

STAGES OF REHABILITATION

(1) Preparing for resettlement (in hospital or community).
(2) Bridging the gap.
(3) Community support.

Preparing for resettlement

Rehabilitation begins with diagnosis. This does not mean that the diagnosis dictates the patient's programme, but rather that, as treatment of the acute illness is initiated, general plans for future management should be discussed. As the acute symptoms subside, more detailed consideration can be given to rehabilitation. The original plans may have to be modified and referral to a special ward or unit focussing on rehabilitation may be considered. For some patients, programmes initiated in hospital may be continued after discharge.

The rehabilitation unit may be a single ward or a comprehensive progressive care system including half-way houses, hostels and group homes attached to the hospital. The patient follows a transitional programme which is designed to reduce dependence on staff and the institution by gradually promoting independence in all aspects of behaviour. Revision of former skills will be required together with re-education for community living. As far as possible, this last phase should take place in accommodation which provides a realistic environment. The ideal final stage is an assessment flat where patients can stay for fixed periods of time to try out their skills with minimal supervision from staff.

Bridging the gap—Resettlement into the community

The rehabilitation process does not end with discharge from hospital. On the contrary, it is intensified as the patient comes face to face with the realities and problems of life in the community. 'Going it alone' and getting to know the locality is a stressful experience for most patients. Support from known and trusted people is essential during this bridging phase if the experiences gained at earlier stages of the programme are to be consolidated and augmented.

Community support

Continuing support will be necessary to maintain progress, provide help at times of crisis and prevent deterioration. For some people day care will be required, while for others the regular supervision of a community nurse or attendance at a medication clinic may suffice.

It is not always recognised that it is possible to become institutionalised in the community just as easily as within hospital.

Support can promote the confidence required to cope with the unexpected events of a rather unstructured existence. This will help prevent the patient from clinging to routines established in hospital which are inappropriate for life outside.

People should be encouraged to make full use of the services and community resources available. They must understand the roles of members of the primary health care team, including the general practitioner, and how to obtain help. The use of lunch clubs and community leisure facilities will continue the development of skills and encourage integration rather than isolation.

The rehabilitation process is summarised in Table 4.1.

TREATMENT PLANNING

Any rehabilitation programme must be based on an assessment of the individual's skills and limitations so that realistic goals may be defined and the appropriate treatment programme devised (Fig. 4.1). Reassessment and evaluation lead

Table 4.1 The rehabilitation process

	Acute Ward	Rehabilitation facility	Community
Task	Reduction of 'illness'	Promotion of independence	Maintenance of level of function
Method	Permitting and encouraging decision-making Preservation of roles and independence	Graded progression of responsibility and goals	Monitoring of progress. Crisis intervention

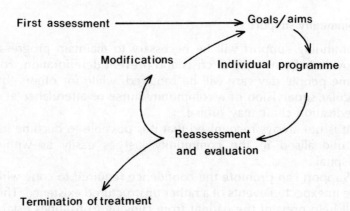

Figure 4.1 The treatment planning cycle.

to modification of the programme and the treatment planning cycle continues. Achievement of a goal allows termination of that particular part of the programme or a change in emphasis. This is discussed in more detail later (Ch. 5).

Gradually, the patient will develop skills and through practice and experience, reach his own level of competence. We must now consider the principles of rehabilitation which form the basis of all treatment planning.

PRINCIPLES OF REHABILITATION—THE THEORY

There is nothing particularly complicated about the theory of rehabilitation. Applying this theory is perhaps not so easy, but then experience is part of any learning process, including rehabilitation itself.

The simple concepts below provide a framework and general approach to the rehabilitation theory: the bricks with which to create structures of any complexity.
Four basic principles are:
(1) Listen to the patient.
(2) Know the community.
(3) Pay attention to detail.
(4) Remember how the world has changed.

Listen to the patient

But of course you do! Remember that it is necessary to listen very carefully to watch the non-verbal messages in order to identify the real problem. It is important to avoid imposing one's own view of the problem on to the patient. Careful open-ended questioning will help the patient to talk about problems which might not have been apparent at first. Other people may have identified all sorts of problems, but it is the individual himself who will tell you what his difficulties really are. However, he may need help separating the core problems from those of less importance.

Know the community

You must be familiar with the community to which your patients are returning if they are to be prepared adequately for the transition. This means not only knowing where to find important local facilities (job centre, health centre, community centre and church), but also how to discover what is available. Members of the rehabilitation team should be aware of directories and resource lists compiled by local councils of social services or mental health groups.

As well as practical information, an understanding of cultural norms is necessary. Your catchment area may include exclusive residential areas, deprived inner city housing estates or ethnic minority groups and you must be aware of 'what goes' in each. Patients moving into unfamiliar surroundings will need guidance about what is expected of them.

There is now increased awareness of transcultural problems, the difficulties experienced by people moving from one country to another. This is not, however, the prerogative of immigrants as moving from a rural community to a city can be just as difficult.

Pay attention to detail

Absolutely nothing is too small or too obvious to be taken for granted. An apparently trivial setback may prove to be an enormous stumbling block for some people. Similarly, routine tasks which most people perform without much thought, for some patients may assume a significance apparently out of all proportion. Just because someone is competent in most aspects of daily living, it is not safe to assume that he can cope with any particular task. It is important to check that he can and to record the result of the observations.

Pat could cook, generally look after himself and coped well at his job in the hospital. A hostel place was found for him on the other side of town. 'No good', he said, 'It's too far to walk.' 'But you can get a bus to the end of the road.' It wasn't just lack of familiarity with the complicated pay-as-you-enter buses, but a hitherto unvoiced delusion had to be considered. Meanwhile, someone else took the bed in the hostel . . .

Remember how the world has changed

For some patients, leaving hospital is like moving to a foreign country with all the anxieties such a change arouses. The feeling of *dis-ease* experienced if one is not *au fait* with social conventions may be shared by a patient who returns home on weekend pass as a virtual stranger visiting his own home.

Changes will be particularly noticeable for long-term patients. They may not even recognise where they used to live with all the new building or the by-pass cutting across town. However, this also has relevance for others. Patterns and norms of society are constantly changing. It does not take long for shops to alter or businesses to move. The micro-chip technology and other developments occur at a bewildering rate, so the adjustments required of our patients multiply. The speed of progress may seem to have alarming dimensions.

The rate of inflation can pose a real problem for patients.

Betty just could not accept that she would have to pay 25p for a pudding to go with the rest of the meal she had so painstakingly selected at the supermarket. She felt she could not possibly justify spending the equivalent of five whole shillings in 'old money'. Indeed, the total of her purchases almost caused her to walk out of the shop empty-handed. Hunger and her escort prevailed upon her to do otherwise!

If all this seems obvious—good! If not, perhaps it has raised questions about your own practice. If you are tempted to by-pass the remainder of the list, remember point 3. Now continue. Further points to consider are:

  (5) Graded programmes
  (6) Timing
  (7) Education and re-education
  (8) Re-orientation
  (9) Staff attitudes
 (10) Consistency
 (11) Security
 (12) Attitudes to medication

Graded programmes

The grading and staging of programmes allows the patient to progress at an individual rate through a series of tasks, towards the achievement of the eventual objective. A goal which seems remote may leave him unmotivated, through lack of conviction that such a task can ever be accomplished. Success in small stages, appropriate to the individual, promotes confidence and will encourage further effort.

Compare the patient's skills to a pile of bricks. To build the wall, bricks are systematically placed in layers to achieve a tall, stable structure. Each brick might be small, but contributes to the finished product. The patient's skills also need to be well integrated and held together on firm foundations.

Timing

One step at a time is enough. The individual needs time to consolidate each new experience before embarking on the next. If, for example, someone has a change of occupation, wait and give him time to adjust to this new routine before making a change in accommodation (unless, of course, circumstances mean that this is impossible or the goals are well within his capabilities). Likewise, medication should not be altered just before a patient moves to a strange unit as he will have enough stress to contend with in the move itself.

Education and re-education

Some people have never had the opportunity to learn basic living skills. Others will have forgotten them, or they may have atrophied through lack of use or illness. Essential skills for each individual will depend on the accommodation anticipated. Someone who aims to live in a hostel may not need to be domestically self-sufficient, whereas no group home resident can survive and co-operate with fellow residents without competence in household tasks. If a patient is unable to reach a safe level of performance, it will be necessary to consider alternative arrangements.

Re-orientation

This is closely linked to 4 and 7. Dormant skills may be renewed in the light of modern requirements. Detailed knowledge of local resources and facilities must be acquired. Some patients have been known to ride a bus from terminus to terminus in order to gain an impression of their new surroundings. Imagine how you would feel moving to a strange town.

Staff attitudes

Attitudes are of paramount importance (see page 55). The role of staff is in some ways similar to that of parent. They provide a secure base from which to experiment and to which to return when in need of succour; but not a dominating influence. Staff may have to learn to stand back and watch a patient struggle to find out things for himself. It is by no means easy to resist the temptation to intervene but allowing impending disaster to materialise may permit valuable learning. Needless to say, success is also necessary and achievements should be reinforced in a way that is not patronising.

Consistency

This is really self-explanatory but conflicting messages and changing attitudes are confusing for patients and staff alike. Firm encouragement one day will be undermined if followed by a *laissez faire* approach the next. Uncertainty about the reaction likely to be received from staff is bound to reduce confidence. Consistency of personnel is as important as consistency of approach. It is inevitable that staff will change and in teaching hospitals, the turnover may be rapid. Newcomers, both staff and patients, take time to settle into the ways of a new unit, and may feel that they are just getting to know the situation when they are moved on again. For the sake of continuity, and to provide a sense of security, it is essential to have a core of permanent staff. This is particularly important in rehabilitation where change may be slow to occur and consistency may be required over several years.

Security

Being able to try something out is the most effective way to learn though not all learning is painless. Patients need an environment in which failure is accepted as part of life, rather than being regarded as a major disaster. They must feel able to accept support and try again.

Patient's attitude to medication

Many people would place this much higher up the list. If a patient cannot appreciate and accept the need for necessary medication, the whole treatment programme may be placed in jeopardy. It can be very hard for some patients to understand the need to take pills, especially when they feel well and have little insight into the fact that they have ever been ill. They may be prepared to swallow medication when supervised, but not when left to their own devices. The need to take a tablet to suppress undesirable side-effects may be more readily understood.

Long-term medication can be hard to accept and the idea of long-term psychotropic medication may lead to the same sort of reactions as are produced by the prospect of insulin or thyroid replacement therapy.

On the other hand, some patients learn to recognise changes in their illness and adjust the medication accordingly.

To turn the rehabilitation process into a working model, the theory requires to be applied throughout all stages of the patient's programme. Caplan stated that 'Rehabilitation begins with diagnosis' and the sooner the process can be started, the greater the chance of prevention of handicap.

THE TREATMENT TEAM

The team is the cornerstone of the rehabilitation process (Ch. 9). Without effective team-work, communication and co-operation, the concepts described above will be of little use. Co-ordination may appear time-consuming, but it is time well invested. Efficient and effective organisation and communication go a long way towards achieving results. The idea of team-work is not idealistic or unattainable but worth working for.

FACTORS INFLUENCING THE REHABILITATION PROCESS

Theory alone is not enough. Staff must be aware of the dynamics of the therapeutic relationship and the factors that will influence this (Fig. 4.2).

Communication

It is crucial to a therapeutic relationship that patients, staff and relatives are clear about the targets to be aimed at and the methods by which they may be achieved. Polak asked newly admitted patients, their relatives, charge nurses and psychiatrists why the patient had been admitted to hospital and what was to be achieved. He found that all the people involved had very different ideas and had assumed that everyone agreed with their viewpoint.

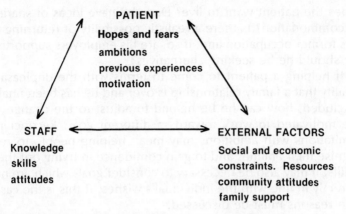

Figure 4.2 Factors influencing the therapeutic relationship.

Good communication with regular review of goals and re-inforcement of achievements will lead to increased motivation on both sides.

It is worth considering our own individual styles of communication. Is the language we use fully understood by the patient? This does not just mean do we speak the same tongue, but is the pattern of speech too complex, are the words used unfamiliar to the social and educational background from which the patient comes? If he is familiar with psychiatric terminology, is his use of words based on genuine understanding or mere repetition of jargon? We may falsely assume that he understands more than he does. Has the communication been two-way? (Try reading Michel Quoist's *The Telephone*.)

All this may sound obvious, but how many people leave their doctor's surgery, sure that they know what has been said, only to wonder some time later what he really meant?

The patient

'You can only rehabilitate a volunteer'. But how is motivation achieved? There is no simple answer. Good communication may facilitate motivation but, of equal importance, is the recognition of the patient's hopes and ambitions. For instance, is discharge an idea which is too remote to be contemplated or a suggestion which is too threatening at present? Where does the patient want to live? Does he have ideas of sharing accommodation? Is there a realistic possibility of returning to his former occupation and, if so, are his employers supportive or should he be seeking alternatives?

If helping a patient to come to terms with the unpleasant reality that a family relationship is over and he has been finally excluded, how can he be helped to adjust to the change or be motivated to work towards a different goal? Reconciling limitations with ambitions may mean helping people to recognise their abilities and to gain confidence in trying out their skills. It may also be necessary to consider goals which are not directly in line with the individual's wishes. If this is the case, the reasons must be discussed.

The staff—knowledge, skills, attitudes

Knowledge

All members of the treatment team will already have some knowledge of psychiatric disorders, consequent problems and their management. In addition to the recognition of illness and its management (physical, medical and social), team members should be aware of the factors contributing to institutionalisation and its prevention (Ch. 2).

The extent and range of any team member's knowledge will depend on the level of training and professional experience. The strength of a clinical team depends on the depth and breadth of experience, both professional and personal, that individuals contribute to the team as a whole. The recognition of each team member's particular areas of knowledge and expertise is vital to the most effective functioning of the team. Which team member knows most about voluntary resources for the elderly? Who enjoys encouraging the patient to take part in social activities? (See Ch. 9)

Skills

Each member of the team will contribute the skills specific to his own professional training: conceptual, diagnostic, organisational, caring and administrative. Some skills will be shared by all team members; skills of listening and observing, and interpersonal relationship skills with the ability to facilitate therapeutic interaction. Of special importance are the skills of counsellor, the ability to provide acceptance, warmth and accurate empathy together with consistency. The focus should be helping the patient to work through problems and identify solutions. It is a necessary part of rehabilitation for him to develop decision-making skills rather than to be told what to do. The temptation to advise or even to dictate may at times be great, but in the long run is counterproductive. Life in hospital may not offer many opportunities for making choices, even in mundane matters.

Leadership skills should be acquired by most members of the team. Any group work with patients requires sensitive leadership. Senior staff will be expected to provide leadership in staff meetings even though planning will be a shared task. The ability to talk through opposing views, to accept the majority view even though it was not one's first choice and to identify particular problems between staff will only come with experience.

Attitudes

Not everyone is suited to the demands of working with rehabilitation patients. The pace is often slow with change occurring over years rather than weeks. Staff must be able to maintain a positive, patient and consistent approach over long periods of time. They must be accepting of the constraints of the illness and of the patient's limitations, even when things go wrong. They must be empathic, being able to understand just what the individual is going through, and must be able to communicate this to the patient.

Above all, a commonsense approach is required. For much of the time, psychiatry will have to be forgotten and all members of the clinical team will have to turn their attention to such practical subjects as how to help the patient undertake a shopping expedition or look after his personal hygiene. Many health care workers are very caring people and it is difficult for them to maintain the correct balance between caring and over-protection.

At times of frustration, disappoinment or failure, it can be hard to maintain therapeutic optimism. It is then that the team must offer each other mutual support and encouragement to avoid being overwhelmed by a sense of hopelessness.

Social, economic and other external influences

Changes in society inevitably affect the task of rehabilitation both directly and indirectly. Economic recession and financial restraints lead to reduced staffing levels and cut-backs in building programmes, both of which can affect staff morale. Faced with the prospect of fewer staff and therefore less time to spend with patients and little prospect of new hostels or facilities being provided, there is a danger that staff 'give up' and rehabilitation slows down. Yet the response can be more creative. If we are unable to provide the same service as before, then we must evaluate which parts of our service are most effective, where is there overlap in what is being provided and decide whether there is a new way of providing something rather different.

At times of mass unemployment, the focus of rehabilitation must change. There is little point in rehabilitating patients for a return to work if no jobs are available. The emphasis must shift to ensuring a good quality of life by providing interests and opportunities apart from work.

Finally, the fact remains that there is a stigma attached to psychiatric illness both for sufferers and those involved in caring for the psychiatrically ill. This will not change without better public understanding of psychiatric disorder.

SUMMARY OF THE PRINCIPLES OF REHABILITATION*

(1) The focus of rehabilitation is the quality of a patient's life, how he or she lives and works.

(2) Commitment to clients is for as long as they want, maybe a lifetime. Our task is to help them make the most of the rest of their lives.

(3) Concentration on the *abilities* of the client and not the *disabilities* to find what skills and what wishes the client has

---

* Adapted from *The Lancet* with the permission of the editor and Dr. David Clark.

in order to build on them rather than drearily to discuss hallucinations.

(4) Challenges can be more valuable to the client than tender loving care and we must judge when reality confrontation will help more than either compassion or medication.

(5) The approach must be multi-disciplinary. No one profession has all the answers to rehabilitation and other patients can often be the individiual's most important source of strength. We have to work towards maximising the patient's social support.

(6) The organisation must be constantly reviewed, attempting to clarify shifting responsibilities. Attention must be paid to larger organisations of which we are a part and to the community we serve.

(7) Research should be a part of rehabilitation.

REFERENCES

Anthony W 1980 The principles of psychiatric rehabilitation. University Park Press, Baltimore
Caplan G 1964 Principles of preventive psychiatry. Basic Books Inc., New York
Cheadle J, Morgan R 1981 Psychiatric rehabilitation. National Schizophrenia Fellowship, 78 Victoria Road, Surbiton, Surrey
Clark D H 1984 The development of a psychiatric rehabilitation service. Lancet 2: 625–627
Garland M 1983 The other side of psychiatric care. Macmillan, London
Hume C A, Pullen I M 1979 Rehabilitation in psychiatry. British Journal of Occupational Therapy 42: 283–285
McCreadie R 1982 Rehabilitation in psychiatric practice. Pitman, London
Quoist M 1963 Prayers of life. Gill and Son, Dublin, p. 15
Shepherd G 1984 Institutional care and rehabilitation. Longman Applied Psychology, London
Watts F, Bennett D (Eds) 1981 Principles of psychiatric rehabilitation. Wiley, Chichester
Willson M 1983 Occupational therapy in long term psychiatry. Churchill Livingstone, Edinburgh
Wing J K, Brown G W 1971 Institutionalism and schizophrenia. Cambridge University Press, Cambridge
Wing J K, Morris B (Eds) 1981 Handbook of psychiatric rehabilitation practice. Oxford University Press, Oxford

The beginning of an acquaintance whether with persons or things is to get a definite outline for our ignorance.

George Eliot, **Daniel Deronda**

5

Introduction to assessment and treatment planning

Clephane Hume

Assessment is the foundation of any treatment regime. The purpose is to provide:

(1) objective rather than anecdotal information;
(2) a measure of skills, achievements, deficits, problems;
(3) a base line from which to monitor change;
(4) standard information, so that groups of patients can be compared for evaluation.

Observations must be carefully recorded so that the information collected is readily available to all members of the treatment team.

ASSESSMENT—METHOD

Most assessments involve observation of patients performing particular tasks. The context may be formal, in that the patient is instructed to carry out specific tasks, or informal, where he is observed over a longer period of time without special instruction. The patient may be involved in self-assessment through the use of questionnaires and inventories.

Assessment skills are not the prerogative of any one profession and should be developed by all members of the team. Many people do observe patients on a day-to-day basis automatically without reflecting too much about this aspect of their work. It is easy to form clinical impressions from these observations but careful recording may reveal a different picture. It is not that most people lack powers of observation, but rather that the difficulty lies in interpretation. Experience and discussion with others involved in patient assessment will help develop these skills.

Recent technological developments have increased the range of assessment media available. Audio and video recorders and computers add to the range and type of material that can be recorded.

Schedules, questionnaires, inventories and check lists

These are all ways of collecting information in a systematic and standard way. The most simple can be administered with little or no training, while the more complex will require special training (e.g. PSE). Specific rehabilitation schedules are available such as the Morningside Rehabilitation Status Scale (Affleck and McGuire, 1984). The testing and interpretation of certain aspects of behaviour or function may be the province of particular members of the team (e.g. I.Q. testing by clinical psychologists).

Standardised interview schedules such as the Present State Examination (PSE) provide detailed, standardised information about the patient and offer useful research data. Computer programs are available to provide a standard diagnosis (e.g. Catego). Computer interviews may become a routine part of assessment as there is some evidence that patients may give more honest answers to a machine than to another, potentially critical, person.

Questionnaires and inventories may be used to gather data for research and evaluation of treatment and progress. They may be completed by staff as part of a standard interview or filled in by the patient to obtain a subjective view of ability.

Graphic scales may be used for observer- or self-assessment. A cross is drawn on a 10 cm line to represent just how the patient is feeling or behaving.

Forms

Although standardised schedules have the advantage of allowing comparison with other units, the team may wish to

devise its own assessment schedule to meet local requirements. Design is important. Any bias on the part of the person
completing the assessment should be minimised by careful
planning and testing, and the information collected must be
clearly recorded without ambiguity. A team wishing to design
its own schedule is advised to seek the advice of a clinical
psychologist in order to avoid well-known pitfalls.

The usual stages are (1) decide on the area to be assessed
(e.g. ability to live on his own), (2) list the topics to be
included (shopping, cooking, budgeting, etc), (3) decide how
it is to be rated and recorded, and (4) try it out. A small pilot
study will inevitably show up problems (e.g. the criteria are
not as clear as was originally thought) and modifications will
be necessary. When all team members can agree on the
scores for particular individuals (inter-rater reliability), the
form is ready for use.

Rating scales of various degrees of complexity may be used.
However, the more gradations in the scale, the less reliable
ratings become and so elaborate gradations are not recommended. It should also be remembered that raters may
develop a fixed way of responding such as avoiding the
extremes of a scale or always rating at the left-hand end of a
scale. The most simple yes/no rating may be sufficient:

    e.g. Can cannot not applicable

          yes yes with difficulty no not applicable

          yes yes with help no not applicable

Alternatively, the rater may have a choice of descriptions,
picking the most applicable (Fig. 5.1).

Adjective	inclines to	average	inclines to	adjective
sad	√			happy
tidy			√	untidy

Figure 5.1 Behaviour rating scale.

The problem with this type of scale is defining what
'frequently' or 'occasionally' mean.

Check-lists may be drawn up to ensure that all relevant
aspects are assessed.

Charts

Charts, such as the Gunzburg PAC (patient assessment chart) present comprehensive information in an easy to read form. A simple pie chart or histogram, which can be filled in when the patient reaches a predetermined stage of rehabilitation, will quickly provide information about areas of achievement and deficit, which means more to most people than particular scores or figures (Fig. 5.2).

Information which is clearly presented and easily understood (preferably on one side of a piece of paper) is much more likely to be used than a dossier of information which is poorly presented and difficult to sort out.

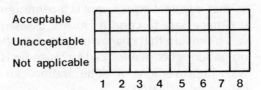

Initial assessment   **Acceptable**

1. Hygiene   **Unacceptable**
2. Budgeting
3. Social interaction   **Not applicable**
4. Time keeping
5. Tidiness
6. Work routine
7. Active symptoms
8. Safety (smoking)

   1 2 3 4 5 6 7 8

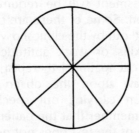

Shade in areas of function in which patient performs adequately. (Gaps identify need for further training.)

Figure 5.2 Recording charts.

ASSESSMENT

When?

Question—When should assessment be carried out?
Answer—At all stages of the programme!

Screening

On referral to a rehabilitation unit, the patient's suitability for admission will be assessed by the team. This screening (see also Chapter 8) should provide the team with sufficient information on which to base their decisions regarding selection of patients for that particular unit.

Initial assessment

After admission and following a suitable interval during which the patient can be familiarised with the routine of the unit, an initial assessment should be carried out. This will serve the dual purpose of recording abilities at the start of the rehabilitation programme as well as providing information for treatment planning.

Of course, staff are constantly observing patients' behaviour so that informal assessment is a continuing process. However, it is necessary to conduct formal assessment at regular intervals to ensure that change is systematically monitored and that no patient gets overlooked because he is unobtrusive. In this way, improvement or deterioration can be clearly seen and causes investigated.

Specific assessment will be required for certain defined areas of function. Some of these are psychological tests (e.g. IQ) to be carried out by the clinical psychologist. Others, such as domestic skills or work aptitude, are traditionally the domain of the occupational therapist, although such assessments will draw upon the observations of other team members. When carrying out specific assessments, it is important to remember that the patient's ability to perform a task at the time of the test does not necessarily mean that he will be motivated to perform that task when left to his own devices. For example, under test conditions, a patient may go shopping and cook a meal but remain poorly motivated to do this following discharge. Observation over a longer period of time will give more accurate information than can be gained from a single exercise. Similarly, the circumstances of assessment must be noted. In respect of domestic assessments, a patient is at a disadvantage in a strange kitchen so that if at all possible, familiar surroundings, ideally home, should be used.

Further selection of patients for specific treatments such as suitability for psychotherapy, reality orientation or social skills training may be indicated. Group leaders will have their own criteria for selection and team members should familiarise themselves with these in order to avoid unrealistic referrals.

As treatment progresses, and if discharge seems feasible, a home visit is indicated. Assessing the individual in familiar surroundings is of immense value and may result in a picture very different from that obtained in the ward.

Pre-discharge assessment

When discharge is imminent, the pre-discharge assessment should provide a summary of current performance. These results may be compared with the initial assessment to show general progress and to evaluate the efficacy of treatment. Alternatively the data may be used as a part of research into the skills needed for living and surviving in the community. This latter relates to the identification of behaviours which will predict the outcome of treatment.

The prime purpose of all the assessments mentioned above is to help the clinical team to provide the best possible treatment and most suitable plans for a particular patient. However, the patient himself should not be excluded. The opportunity should always be taken to discuss the findings with the patient, even if only in the most general terms. This feedback allows some reality testing and learning to occur. The formal recognition of progress will be useful to those with low self-esteem and an accurate assessment will be of help to those who are over-confident or unrealistic in their view of themselves.

ASSESSMENT

Of what?

There is an infinite number of answers to this particular question. The choice of assessment must be tailored to the individual case. Some examples are given to illustrate common topics.

(1) Mental state: appearance and behaviour, speech, thoughts, mood, cognitive function, memory.

(2) Cognitive function: comprehension, memory, decision-making, orientation.

(3) Personal care: hygiene, appearance, clothing, use of appliances (teeth, spectacles, etc).

(4) Social skills: interpersonal relationships, communication patterns, telephoning, literacy, advice-seeking and giving, non-verbal skills, assertive behaviour.

(5) Domestic skills: laundry, meal planning and preparation, household cleaning and management, security and safety, dealing with emergencies.

(6) Leisure: hobbies, interests, friends, participation in activities.

(7) Work: general work habits, aptitudes, attitudes, ambitions, job seeking skills, relationships.

(8) Community skills: mobility, use of transport, road safety, orientation, local knowledge.

(9) Home visit: facilities available, level of support, evidence of previous coping or non-coping.

Interpretation

To be of use, the findings of assessment and their significance must be interpreted accurately according to individual circumstances. For example, in a hospital assessment of domestic skills, one patient complained that he could not make his bed as the blankets were 'too difficult'. It was only later discovered that at home he used a continental quilt and so the problem was not what it originally seemed to be. In fact he now manages quite independently.

TREATMENT PLANNING

Treatment planning, like assessment, must be seen as a continuous process. The initial plan is only the starting point. The absence of clear goals and identifiable steps towards achieving them leads to confusion and loss of interest. The patient will not remain motivated if he is unsure of his goals and staff lose enthusiasm if there is no clear target.

What is the target?

Defining targets and goals can only start after an assessment of the situation has been made. With a base-line which indicates the achievements and deficits of the individual, there is a starting point for working out short-term and long-term goals, and how they are to be achieved.

The patient may have his own clear goals in mind, such as getting a job or staying in hospital. The team may consider the patient a candidate for a group home or for a sheltered job. Staff and patients must discuss and agree on the aims, the order in which they are to be tackled and just how they may be achieved.

Although the overall aim of a treatment plan may be a significant change in the patient's lifestyle (for example, discharge from hospital to a flat of his own), it is essential that the steps on the way to achieving this goal are of a size which the patient thinks are possible. Staged goals must be set in the context of a general plan which cannot be restricted to the confines of the rehabilitation unit. It may be important to involve family and friends at the planning stage.

Deciding on specific goals may be carried out on an individual contractual basis or in a group where weekly targets are set and discussed by the members. While staff may have preliminary discussions, the patient should always be included in the decision-making process.

Recording the treatment plan and goals

Information regarding the goals for each patient must be readily available to the team. Use of a problem-oriented approach, such as the nursing care plan or problem-oriented medical records, provides clear information about the goals, the proposed action to be taken and who in the team will be primarily responsible for each task. This type of approach also has the benefit of maintaining a record of problems which have already been dealt with (Fig. 5.3).

While individual team members will have separate tasks on which to work with the patient, it is important that all team members are clear about this so that conflicts or duplication of effort do not occur (See Ch. 9). These only serve to frustrate patients and staff, are detrimental to team relationships and are easily avoided by effective communication. Efficient record-keeping is also helpful to new members of staff,

NAME	UNIT		
problem	action	by whom	outcome
Using public transport (Wants to visit brother)	1. Discuss what is involved	S. Maclean	Can identify bus number, stops and describe procedure
	2. Go into town for tea.	S. Maclean	
	3. Travel alone	Check "	
	4. Visit brother	Check "	
Dentures not fitting	Refer to dentist	K. Reid	Appointment made for 28th May, 10 am

Figure 5.3 Example of problem-oriented records.

including students, who can readily find out what the aims are for any particular patient.

Verbal reports at meetings are essential for quick communication but must be backed up with written confirmation. This will provide a permanent record for future reference and can be referred to by members not present at that particular meeting. It is worth considering how teams operate. If you miss a weekly review meeting, how do you find out what decisions have been made? If a team member is absent, how do you find out what has already been done?

Implementing a treatment plan

The construction of a problem list may prove to be a great deal easier than implementing the proposed treatment plan. Apparently simple targets may require a great deal of work to implement. Progress may be facilitated by sub-dividing and grading the tasks. Initially smaller and easier tasks can be tackled, progressing towards the major hurdles. Activity analysis, the analysis of the component parts to any task, may be helpful. Take the apparently simple task of scrambling an egg and imagine teaching it to someone who has never done it before. Writing a step-by-step guide involves an amazing number of operations.

The order in which tasks are tackled will be important. Shopping is not the recommended way to start a domestic skills programme. Some simple tasks such as making tea and toast will provide an assessment of competence and general kitchen knowledge. Next, discussion and planning of a straightforward meal will lead on to the preparation of a shopping list, including the quantities required. The location of the shops should be identified, financial arrangements made and, if transport is necessary, details worked out. Then, and only then, should shopping be tackled.

Evaluation of individual programmes

The continuing nature of the treatment planning process requires that results should be constantly evaluated. If the assessments show that a particular goal has been mastered, then treatment may shift to the next goal. Sometimes a goal will not be achieved and modification and alteration of aims may be required. The new plan will in turn be evaluated so that further modifications can be implemented.

Evaluation of the treatment approach

Just as it is necessary constantly to evaluate and modify treatment plans for an individual, it is equally important to consider the emphasis of the rehabilitation unit programmes. Social changes, such as rising unemployment, may render previous goals invalid. For a group of patients unlikely to find work in a climate of high unemployment, the emphasis should shift away from training for work towards training for leisure.

Evaluation should also include consideration of the treatment environment (Moos, 1974).

REFERENCES

Affleck J W, McGuire R S 1984 The measurement of psychiatric rehabilitation status—a review of the needs and a new scale. British Journal of Psychiatry 145:517
Clark D H 1981 Social therapy in psychiatry, 2nd edn. Churchill Livingstone, Edinburgh
Cochrane R 1983 The social creation of mental illness. Longman Applied Psychology, London
Gunzburg H C 1973 Social competence and mental handicap, 2nd edn. Balliere Tindall, London

Moos R 1974 Evaluating treatment environments. J Wiley, New York

Mosey A C 1973 Activities therapy. Raven Press, New York

Peck D, Dean C 1983 In: Kendell R, Zealley A (eds) Companion to psychiatric studies, 3rd edn. Churchill Livingstone, Edinburgh

Shepherd G 1984 Institutional care and rehabilitation. Longman Applied Psychology, London

Weed L L 1969 Medical records, medical education and patient care. Press of Case Western Reserve University, Cleveland

Willson M 1983 Occupational therapy in long term psychiatry. Churchill Livingstone, Edinburgh

Wing J K, Morris B 1981 Handbook of psychiatric rehabilitation practice. Oxford University Press, Oxford

Patients may recover in spite of drugs or because of them.

J H Gaddum, 1959

6

Treatment

Ian Pullen

Treatment planning is the key to successful rehabilitation (See Ch. 5).

It is part of the standard procedure of:
(1) Assessment
(2) Diagnosis—nosological
             formulation
             problem list
(3) Treatment—physical   } includes where, expected
             social   } effects, duration, review
             psychological } date.
(4) Review—modification of plans

This logical procedure should be followed in all cases. A diagnosis cannot be made without taking a full psychiatric history and mental state examination. There are no short cuts. A nosological diagnosis (assigning the patient to a particular diagnostic group, e.g. schizophrenia) and a formulation (an explanation of why the patient has developed this particular illness or has relapsed at this particular time) are required. Further assessment may be required to arrive at a full problem list.

Treatment plans must include: whether treatment of any type is required or is likely to help; where treatment should be carried out; the form, duration and expected effects as

69

well as likely side-effects; whether the patient is able to give informed consent and, if not, whether the treatment should be compulsory. Treatments may be used separately or in combination.

A review date should be set and necessary changes made.

PROBLEMS FOR REHABILITATION

The long term rehabilitation group of patients present particular problems in terms of treatment. They suffer from chronic conditions which require treatment over long periods of time, in some cases for life. It is easy to lose sight of the treatment goals and the rationale behind the treatment chosen. In desperation, drug doses may be pushed up to unacceptable levels and unhelpful combinations used. Some patients change little, if at all, despite the various treatments tried but may develop irreversible changes due to long-term exposure to medication (such as tardive dyskinesia or hypothyroidism).

Many patients may be suitable for rehabilitation and resettlement, but still have only minimal insight into the fact that they have been ill. With these patients motivation and compliance may prove to be problems.

MODELS OF MENTAL ILLNESS

At our present state of knowledge there are many different ways of conceptualising any particular patient's condition. The model chosen may depend on training, dogma, or an eclectic use of the model that best suits that particular patient. The significance for this discussion is that the model chosen will dictate the treatment to be used.

The most important models are: organic, psychotherapeutic, behavioural, social and medical. Other models include the conspiratorial, family interaction and moral models (See Clare).

(1) Organic model

This model considers all psychiatric symptoms to be the result of some underlying physical condition. The acute confusional state produced by a serious infection such as pneumonia, and the mood disturbances brought about by the hormone abnormalities of thyroid and pituitary disease are such conditions. There is certainly a growing list of conditions for which an organic cause has been found, but few psychiatrists would claim that all psychiatric illness can be explained in this way.

(2) Psychotherapeutic model

This model stresses the importance of early childhood experience in the emergence later in life of psychiatric conditions. Failure to master vital developmental hurdles may lead to a re-emergence, under stress, of the emotional and relationship difficulties of an earlier stage of life. These unconscious mechanisms include fixation and regression. While these theories may aid the understanding of neuroses, there is, as yet, little objective evidence to show that psychotherapeutic measures are effective.

(3) Behavioural approach

Learning theory suggests that all behaviour is learned. Behaviour that produces pleasurable responses tends to be repeated (reinforced), while behaviour that is linked with a less pleasurable outcome is not repeated (extinguished). Behaviourists deny the existence of the 'unconscious'. Phobias and obsessions have been successfully treated along these lines.

(4) Social model

The social model widens the area of psychiatric involvement. Unlike the previous models which are concerned with the individual, this model includes the individual plus his social situation within the remit of psychiatric interest. Labelling and the concepts of primary and secondary deviance are introduced. Deviant behaviour (Primary deviance) may lead to a person being labelled as mentally ill. Being treated as mentally ill and admitted to hospital may cause abnormal behaviour (Secondary deviance). The social model of psychiatric illness has encouraged such developments as the therapeutic community.

(5) Medical model

The medical model takes into account not merely the symptom, syndrome or disease, but the person who suffers, his personal and social situation, his biological, psychological, and social status. The medical model, as applied to psychiatry, embodies the basic principle that every illness is the product of two factors: environment working on the organism (Clare). Thus the medical model is not to be confused, as it often is, with the narrow organic model.

Purists insist that only one model should be used. Yet, at present, no one model can explain all psychiatric conditions any more than any single method of treatment has been found that is universally effective.

In rehabilitation a flexible approach is recommended based on the medical model, but using other models where applicable. There may well be occasions where two different treatment approaches, based on different models, may be used simultaneously. Thus a man being resettled after developing schizophrenia may receive medication (medical model) in a hostel run on therapeutic community lines (social model) while receiving social skills training (behavioural model). At the end of the day we are all in the business of doing the best for our patients rather than proving that our ideological stance is best.

VARIETIES OF TREATMENT

Environmental context will suggest the treatments most suitable. As most treatments can be applied in any setting, the decision where to treat the patient should be based on social, rather than strictly medical criteria. (See Ch. 3.)

Choice of treatment

In addition to the factors mentioned above, the duration of the illness will have to be considered. Is this an acute illness, is it chronic, or is it an acute episode in a chronic condition?

Table 6.1 Choice of treatment

Illness	Problems	Treatment
Acute psychosis	? precipitants, identify stresses, where to treat, ? medication	likely to include short-term medication plus social intervention
Chronic psychosis	continuing stresses rehabilitation, compliance and motivation	? depot medication behaviour therapy, social therapies
Acute or chronic	precipitants ? stopped medication	? depot medication long-term, move to a hostel or other environmental manipulation

PHYSICAL METHODS OF TREATMENT

Physical methods of treatment are used as part of an overall plan. There are clear indications for their use in treatment rather than merely for 'patient control'.

Psychotropic drugs

A number of simple guidelines ensure the sensible and safe use of medication. These may be summarised as:

specific indications	—e.g. diagnosis
use well-tried drugs	—the newest might not be the best
dose	—may be crucial to be effective
	—special care in elderly
frequency/route of administration	—may affect compliance
? contraindications	—drug interaction
set date for review	—review short-term medication at least weekly, long-term monthly
monitor	—response/side effects/toxic effects
use drugs singly	—avoid two drugs of same type
	—avoid drugs to mask side-effects

if no change   —check compliance, consider whether further drugs justified

who prescribes   —must be clear, GP or hospital

These recommendations represent a common-sense approach which is clear and easy to apply. However, the rehabilitation and long-stay populations present management problems which sometimes provoke a muddled response. It is not unusual to find long-stay patients on a number of different drugs of the same group (perhaps three major tranquillisers), very high dosage with drugs to counteract side-effects and, at the same time, a clear statement in the medical notes to the effect that 'this patient has not responded to any medication'.

Another common pattern is for a disturbed patient to receive a relatively high dose of medication quite appropriately. Then, as the patient settles, staff anxieties resist the idea of drug reduction 'in case he relapses'. When a relapse does occur the drugs are again increased. The pattern repeats itself and soon the patient is receiving very high doses of medication.

Sensible prescribing requires knowledge of the mode and duration of action of drugs (half-life). Drugs should be prescribed to be taken as few times a day as possible as this will encourage compliance and also prevent accumulation of the drug. Thus some drugs must be given four hourly (droperidol) while others only monthly (depot haloperidol).

Not only is it bad practice to give a second drug to counteract the side effects of the first drug, but, in some cases, it is dangerous. It is now known that the routine prescription of 'anti-parkinson' medication with major tranquillisers may increase the risk of the patient developing irreversible tardive dyskinesia (involuntary movements). Good prescribing means considering carefully the short and long term effects of any course of action.

Full prescribing information is given in standard textbooks. A small selection of common drugs, such as any doctor might normally use, is given here (Table 6.2).

Sometimes it is difficult for non-medical staff to understand why a particular drug has been selected from within a group.

Table 6.2 A short list of psychotropic drugs

Major tranquillisers	Antidepressants	Minor tranquillisers (night sedation)
Chlorpromazine	Amitriptyline	Diazepam
Thioridazine	Imipramine	
Trifluoperazine		Temazepam
	Mianserin	
Haloperidol		
Depot preparations:		
Fluphenazine decanoate	M.A.O.I.	
Flupenthizol decanoate	Phenelzine	
Haloperidol decanoate		

Others: Lithium carbonate

The choice will depend more on the doctor's familiarity with the drug than specific indications. In fact there is little to chose between most of the drugs within a group. For example, all of the tricyclic antidepressants appear to be equally effective although some may be rather more sedating (Amitriptyline) than others (Imipramine).

ECT (electroconvulsive therapy)

In recent years much has been written about ECT, both for and against. Often the articles in the press have been written in emotive terms, describing the treatment as barbaric and used as punishment. The objective evidence is presented clearly by Clare (1980).

The generally accepted view, in Britain, is that ECT is an effective and safe treatment for severe depression with biological features (early morning wakening, weight loss, delusions). It may also be used in severe mania which is unresponsive to drug treatment. The role of ECT in schizophrenia is much more contentious, and probably most British psychiatrists consider that it should not be used.

The patient should have the procedure explained and reasons for choosing this treatment discussed. He should then be in a position to give informed consent for treatment to proceed. Some patients may be incapable of giving informed consent either because they are too ill to understand the discussion fully, or because their decision would be made on the basis of their delusions. In either case a second, independent consultant opinion is required. The situation regarding compulsory patients is discussed below.

ECT is administered to the anaesthetised and muscle-relaxed patients once or twice a week for an average of four to eight treatments. (A brief description of how to give ECT is given by Cramer et al, 1982.) It may be given simultaneously with antidepressant medication. As with other treatments the treatment should be regularly reviewed.

Psychosurgery

In 1936 Moniz described the first 20 cases treated by interrupting the connections between the frontal lobes and the 'emotion regulating centres' of the subcortical areas of the brain. At first he used alcohol injection, but later used a surgical knife called a leucotome. This treatment and its later refinements gained rapid popularity. Moniz was jointly awarded the Nobel Prize for Physiology and Medicine in 1949. Reaching its peak in the mid 1950s, psychosurgery was aimed at the frontal lobes for anxiety and depression, and the cingulate gyrus for aggression and obsessional disorders.

Between 1942 and 1954, 10 365 people underwent leucotomy for serious mental illness in Britain. Two-thirds of the patients were chronic schizophrenics. The number now is probably less than 100 a year. It is sad that a treatment to which so many patients have been exposed has not been adequately investigated by the usual controlled trials. In Britain it is now seldom considered. It has never been considered to be very effective in schizophrenia and so, except in the most exceptional circumstances, it seems unlikely that readers of this book are likely to look after a patient receiving this treatment.

Psychotherapy

Psychotherapy is any form of 'talking cure' (Rycroft, 1972). It may be interpretive, supportive or behavioural (See Ch. 8), superficial or deep, and individual or group. In Britain, psychotherapy tends to be used with patients suffering from neurosis or a mild degree of personality disorder. Its role in other conditions is contentious.

In the United States it has been the practice to treat schizophrenic patients with both drugs and psychotherapy and some psychiatrists consider psychotherapy to be the treatment of choice (Karon and Vandenbos, 1981). This is discussed in more detail later.

Social treatment

Many psychiatric conditions are precipitated by stress and the functional psychoses (manic-depressive illness and schizophrenia) are thought to result from the interplay of an inherited tendency and stress. Social treatments are aimed at reducing the level of stress in the lives of patients at risk of relapse. These interventions include education, changing the behaviour of relatives and reducing the amount of time that the patient and relatives spend together. These treatments are still in the experimental stage but early reports are encouraging.

Taking schizophrenia as the model, aetiology, the rationale for treatment and practical treatment arrangements will be discussed.

SCHIZOPHRENIA

About one per cent of the population of the Western world suffer from schizophrenia, the peak incidence occurring between 25–30 years of age. Similar rates have been found in all cultures.

Schizophrenic patients are not equally distributed throughout the country, but tend to be over-represented in run-down city centres. At first this was thought to be due to the 'schizophrenogenic' effect of city life (the breeder theory). But now it is recognised that the illness leads to loss of social competence and earning power and those patients not supported by their family drift to cheaper areas (drift theory).

Diagnosis

The diagnosis of schizophrenia relies on the clinical examination: history and mental state examination. There is no specific diagnostic test available. The ICD-9 (International

Classification of Diseases—Ch. 2) provides a glossary which allows the diagnosis to be made in descriptive terms.

Schizophrenia affects personality, thoughts and mood. The major symptoms arise from a failure to recognise boundaries; between self and the environment, and between different thoughts. Thus a failure to recognise where he ends and the world begins means that his own thoughts appear to come from outside him (auditory hallucinations). He is also unable to distinguish one thought from the next.

His train of speech may be interrupted by unrelated sentences being interpolated. In a more severe form of thought disorder a series of apparently unrelated thoughts may be spoken ('knight's move' thinking). In extreme forms a 'word salad' is produced as words from separate ideas are strung together. This flow of words will be totally unintelligible to the listener. Sudden interruptions to the flow of speech (thought blocking) may produce explanatory delusions such as 'The man next door is taking away my thoughts by laser'.

Emotion is also affected. Often blunting of affect (mood) occurs with little or no emotional response and difficulty in making emotional contact or rapport with others. Sometimes the affect is incongruous, that is out of keeping with circumstances. An extreme example would be laughter when a patient was told that his mother had died. This is not a sign of callousness, but disorganisation.

The other aspect of the person to be affected by the schizophrenic process is the personality. The commonly held view of the schizophrenic 'split personality' is erroneous. The personality is shattered, altering drive to produce apathy and unpredictable behaviour.

The range of experiences described as the 'symptoms of the first rank' are given on page 18. These symptoms are only diagnostic of schizophrenia if the content of the delusions and hallucinations is not readily explainable in terms of the prevailing mood, and they occur in full consciousness. Thus a very depressed person who hears two 'voices' talking to each other about him while referring to him in the third person is not schizophrenic, if they talk only about miserable and depressive things. Nor may a patient be diagnosed as schizophrenic if clouding of consciousness is present (delirium or acute confusion).

Aetiology

The causes of schizophrenia are not fully understood. The vulnerability-stress model is useful in understanding onset and relapse. This proposes a mixture of:

Inherited predisposition + environmental stress

Genetic factors

The general population risk of schizophrenia (one per cent) rises to 15 per cent for the offspring of an affected parent. The risk for someone with an affected identical twin (monozygotic) is about 40 per cent compared with 15 per cent for non-identical (dizygotic) twins.

Stress

Acute stress is important in precipitating schizophrenia. There is a higher than average level of stressful life events in the three weeks prior to the onset of the illness (Brown and Birley, 1968). But more chronic stress is also important. Schizophrenic patients discharged home to relatives have a higher relapse rate than those being discharged to live on their own (Brown et al, 1966).

Expressed emotion (EE) is a measure of the number of critical comments made by relatives and the extent of emotional over-involvement and hostility expressed by relatives. This can be assessed by a complex interview (Camberwell Family Interview). A number of studies have found an association between relapse of schizophrenia and the EE of the key relative living with the patient (Brown et al, 1972; Vaughn and Leff, 1976). Patients returning to live with high EE relatives had a higher relapse rate (51 per cent) than those returning to live with low EE relatives (13 per cent). Two factors appear to lessen the effect of high EE relatives: the amount of face-to-face contact with the relative, and medication. Low contact (less than 35 hours per week) and regular medication reduce relapse rate (15 per cent) in the high EE group, while lack of regular medication and high contact with the relative (more than 35 hours per week) greatly increase the relapse rate (92 per cent) (Vaughn and Leff, 1976).

Viruses

There has been recent speculation about whether schizophrenia is catching (Crow, 1983), but the evidence is slender.

Brain structure

CT scans (computer assisted tomography) have demonstrated dilated ventricles in the brains of about 20 per cent of schizophrenics. This change correlates most with the so-called defect state, the type of condition least responsive to drug treatment.

Dopamine theory

Over the years numerous biochemical theories have been proposed to explain schizophrenia. The amine hypothesis implicates dopamine, a chemical transmitter present in the brain, as the most effective drugs (the major tranquillisers) all block dopamine pathways. As yet there is no conclusive evidence.

Schizophrenogenic families

American writers in the 1950s and 60s promulgated the idea of pathological families which produced schizophrenic children, not by inheritance, but by their pathological interactions. Bateson (1956) produced the 'double bind' theory. This suggested that children were turned into schizophrenics by receiving, continually, double and incongruous messages from the parents. They had to respond to both incompatible messages and not comment on them. The double bind is sometimes used in humour: a New York Jewish mother gave her son a red tie and a green tie for his birthday. When next they met he was wearing the green tie. 'So you don't like the red tie,' said his mother. He just couldn't win! The experimental evidence in support of the double bind theory is trivial.

Singer and Wynne (1965) claimed consistent abnormalities of speech in the parents of schizophrenics, but in London Hirsch and Leff (1975) in a blind controlled trial failed to confirm these findings.

As yet there has been no convincing experimental evidence to support the concept of the schizophrenogenic family.

Psychoanalytic theory

Freudian theory considers schizophrenia to be a regression to the early narcissistic level where the child does not distinguish between self and environment—that is loss of object relations. Reviewing the contribution that psychoanalysis has made towards the understanding of schizophrenia, Clare (1980) considers it to be 'far from self-evident'. He adds that it is worth noting that Freud never deliberately attempted to analyse a psychotically ill patient.

TREATMENTS

Physical

Chlorpromazine was introduced in 1953 and rapidly replaced earlier attempts at treatment. There is now overwhelming experimental evidence to support the clinical experience that major tranquillisers are effective.

An American group (NIMH, 1964) studied 463 young schizophrenics during their first or second acute illness. A double blind study of three different phenothiazines and placebo (no treatment) showed that the drugs were all better than placebo, but that there was nothing to chose between the three drugs.

In chronic schizophrenia the response is less dramatic. Caffey et al (1964) studied 350 chronic schizophrenics all of whom had received phenothiazines for some years. The patients were divided into three groups: one group remained on their present medication; the second group had their medication halved; and the third group were transferred to a placebo 'treatment'. At four months five per cent of those patients left on their original medication had relapsed, compared with 15 per cent of the patients on half medication and 45 per cent of those on placebo. In other words the drugs are having a considerable effect even after years, and the doses used were not excessive.

A third and interesting study was conducted in London by Leff and Wing (1971). They screened all admissions to the Maudsley hospital for a 20 month period for schizophrenia (first episode) and who were well six weeks after discharge. They started with 116, but only 35 entered the trial: 15 were considered to be too ill to risk the possibility of placebo treatment; 11 were too well to require any treatment; 24 just dropped out. Of the 35 in the trial 35 per cent of those receiving the drug relapsed within one year compared with 80 per cent of those receiving the placebo. Of great interest was that the investigators also followed up the patients excluded from the trial. Those who were thought too ill did badly on treatment (67 per cent relapse) while those considered too well did indeed do well without treatment (27 per cent relapse). It appears that drugs are most effective in the middle spectrum of the illness.

Psychotherapy

This is commonly used for schizophrenia in the States, but not in Britain. What is the evidence?

May (1968), in California, randomly allocated 228 schizophrenic patients to five treatment groups: phenothiazines; psychotherapy (analytic—two hours per week minimum); phenothiazine + psychotherapy; ECT; and milieu therapy (just on a ward with other patients). The best outcome was equally divided between the phenothiazine group and the phenothiazine + psychotherapy group. Third was the ECT group followed by the psychotherapy and milieu therapy fourth equal. The effect of the psychotherapy, which was the most expensive form of treatment, was undetectable.

Karon and Vandenbos (1981) still claim that psychotherapy is the treatment of choice, but their own experimental design was faulty. For example all of the patients were 'unquestionably schizophrenic' but precise criteria for inclusion are not given. It must be concluded that the case for the treatment of schizophrenia by psychotherapy is, at best, unproven, and probably it is not useful.

Psychosocial interventions

Five controlled studies assessing the effect of psychosocial interventions with families of schizophrenics have been reviewed by Barrowclough and Tarrier (1984). Of these only two were considered to be well designed.

Falloon and colleagues in California randomly assigned 36 patients to 'family therapy' or 'individual therapy'. All were diagnosed as suffering from schizophrenia on Present State Examination (PSE). Most were living with high EE families. The 'family therapy' package included: education about the nature, course and treatment of schizophrenia; the teaching of problem-solving skills for coping with stress, and communication skills training. The control group received individual supportive psychotherapy. Both groups were controlled on medication and had emergency visits and help with finances and accommodation.

Only one patient relapsed in the family treatment group (6 per cent) compared with eight relapses in the individual therapy group (44 per cent) after nine months treatment. After two years, only three of the individually treated group (17 per cent) had not relapsed compared with 15 of the family group (83 per cent).

Leff and colleagues (1982) treated 24 patients selected as being at very high risk of relapse. All had a relative rated as high on EE with whom they were in contact for over 35 hours a week. All received a PSE diagnosis of schizophrenia. The high EE relatives were the target of social intervention: relatives' group to which high and low EE relatives were invited and encouraged to discuss problems of coping; individual family sessions in the relatives' home aimed at reducing EE and/or contact.

At nine months the experimental group had a nine per cent relapse rate (one patient) compared with 50 per cent in the control group (normal outpatient follow up).

Despite these dramatic results they only succeeded in lowering the EE in six out of 12 families, and reducing contact in five out of 12. Although critical comments within the family were reduced, the treatment was less successful in reducing emotional over-involvement.

MANAGEMENT OF SCHIZOPHRENIA

The main problems encountered are:
(1) the negative symptoms: withdrawal, apathy, thought disorder;
(2) the positive symptoms: hallucinations and delusions;
(3) lack of insight and therefore the need for treatment;

(4) periods of acute disturbance;
(5) social, family and work stresses.

Pre-treatment assessment arrives at a firm diagnosis, provides a baseline measure of symptoms, identifies stresses which may have precipitated the illness and may affect recovery, and assesses the prognosis and need for treatment.

Acute treatment

The choice between home, day or hospital care will depend on the severity of symptoms, the facilities available and the support available at home. The family (and patient) will require information: an explanation of the medication to be used, the reason for admission or day hospital attendance and a realistic time-scale for treatment.

Major tranquillisers are commonly used, starting with chlorpromazine 100 mg three times a day. The dose is increased weekly in most cases, but more rapidly in very disturbed patients, up to 1000 mg a day. If side-effects appear, the dose should, if possible, be reduced. If this is impossible because of the severity of the illness, anticholinergic drugs (such as procyclidine) will be required. If the patient refuses medication and is acutely disturbed, compulsory treatment under the Mental Health Acts may be required.

The family and patient will require support. The family's reaction to the illness may be similar to that described for physical disability (Ch. 13). The patient requires personal contact with a limited number of staff in order to build up trust.

Medication may be slowly reduced once a substantial improvement of symptoms has occurred. Excessive drowsiness, akathisia (motor restlessness) and marked stiffness or tremor suggest a further drug reduction. It is advisable not to change drug dosage at the time of discharge from hospital or transfer to day hospital. If the patient remains well for two to three months, drugs may be stopped completely.

The very disturbed patient

Major tranquillisers, given intramuscularly if necessary, may be required in very high doses: chlorpromazine 100–200 mg

IM three to four hourly or haloperidol 10 mg IM or IV three to four hourly. Very occasionally, morphine may be required to control an extremely disturbed patient.

The patient should be nursed in quiet surroundings, preferably in bed, with a nurse in attendance. After a few days, it should be possible to replace the injections by an adequate dose of oral medication. It should be remembered that the reluctant patient might find it more difficult to hide liquid preparations than tablets. Anti-parkinsonian drugs (procyclidine 5–10 mg orally or IM) may be required to cover side-effects especially as the patient improves.

Long-term management

The prognosis of schizophrenia is very variable. Some patients recover completely. Others continue to require medication to suppress their psychotic experiences, while a third group respond only partially, if at all, to medication. The prognostic indicators in schizophrenia are given in Table 6.3.

After a first illness, medication should be stopped following recovery. If the symptoms have failed to respond to treatment after three months, and staff are sure that the patient has received the medication, the treatment should be reviewed. If two or three major tranquillisers have been tried in adequate dosage, there is no point in persisting and drugs should be stopped.

Table 6.3 Prognostic indicators in schizophrenia

Good prognosis
No family history of schizophrenia
Normal pre-morbid personality
Acute onset
Confusion
Precipitating cause
Depression/elation
Onset after age of 30
Married
Early treatment

If the patient is recovering from his second or third illness in a short time—two or three years—or where the illness has been very severe and caused major disruption to his life, maintenance medication should be continued for at least two years. If the patient is co-operative, then oral medication should be used. Compliance may be improved by a once daily preparation (such as trifluoperazine spansules). If the patient is unreliable, or reluctant to take medication, he may agree to the routine of a depot preparation fortnightly (flupenthixol decanoate) or monthly (haloperidol decanoate).

In all cases, regular assessment will be required to monitor change and to enable planning for other aspects of treatment and living situation. The emotional pattern of the family will indicate the suitability of a return home, the need for hostel care or a day placement. In the light of experimental evidence, attempts may be made to change the family's pattern of expressed emotion.

Other medication

The routine prescription of anti-parkinsonian medication to cover the side-effects of major tranquillisers has been called into question by studies suggesting that their routine prescription increases the risk of the patient developing tardive dyskinesia. This unpleasant, sometimes permanent condition produces involuntary writhing and grimacing movements. All patients receiving regular major tranquillisers should be screened for the development of tardive dyskinesia. Small undulations of the tongue within the mouth may be the earliest signs. Later, jerky, writhing movements of the tongue and smacking lip movements are added to involuntary movements of the jaw, face and limbs.

Dose reduction is the first step. About one-third of patients will improve following withdrawal of the major tranquilliser although symptoms may at first get worse. For some patients, whose hallucinations and delusions become more marked on withdrawing the tranquilliser, the choice will have to be made between the possible permanent dyskinesia or the distress of the psychosis.

Other aspects of treatment planning have been considered in Chapter 5.

Other conditions

As schizophrenia is the condition most commonly encountered in rehabilitation work, the research findings on aetiology and treatment have been discussed in some detail. It is beyond the scope of this book to discuss the treatment of other conditions. A growing literature exists and the presentation of a review article to the team may help stimulate discussion about the most logical ways to treat a chronically disabled patient.

REFERENCES

Barrowclough C, Tarrier N 1984 'Psychosocial' interventions with families and their effects on the course of schizophrenia: a review. Psychological Medicine 14: 629–42

Bateson G, Jackson D D, Haley J, Weakland J H 1956 Toward a theory of schizophrenia. Behavioral Science 1: 251–64

Brown G W, Birley J L T 1968 Crises and life changes and the onset of schizophrenia. Journal of Health and Social Behaviour 9: 203–14

Brown G W, Birley J L T, Wing J K 1972 Influence of family life on the course of schizophrenic disorders: a replication. British Journal of Psychiatry 121: 241–58

Brown G W, Bone U, Dalinson B M, Wing J K 1966 Schizophrenia and social care. Oxford University Press, London

Caffey E M, Diamond L S, Frank T V, Grasberg J C, Herman L, Klell C J, Rothstein C 1964 Discontinuation or reduction of chemotherapy in chronic schizophrenics. Journal of Chronic Diseases 17: 347–58

Clare A 1980 Psychiatry in dissent, 2nd edn. Tavistock Publications, London

Crammer J, Barraclough B, Heine B 1982 The use of drugs in psychiatry. Gaskell, London

Crow T J 1983 Is schizophrenia an infections disease? Lancet i: 173–5

Falloon I, Watt D C, Shepherd M 1978 A comparative controlled trial of pimozide and fluphenazine decanoate in the continuation therapy of schizophrenia. Psychological Medicine 8: 59–70

Hirsch S R, Leff J P 1975 Abnormalities in parents of schizophrenics. Maudsley Monograph No. 22, Oxford University Press, London

Karon B P, Vandenbos G R 1981 Psychotherapy of schizophrenia. The treatment of choice. Jason Aponson, New York

Leff J P, Kuipers L, Berkowitz R, Eberlein Vries R, Sturgeon D 1982 A controlled trial of social intervention in the families of schizophrenic patients. British Journal of Psychiatry 141: 121–34

Leff J P, Wing J K 1971 Trial of maintenance therapy in schizophrenia. British Medical Journal iii: 599–604

May P R A 1968 Treatment of schizophrenia: a comparative study of 5 treatment methods. Science House, New York

NIMH (National Institutes of Mental Health) 1964 Phenothiazine treatment in schizophrenia. Archives of General Psychiatry 10: 246–61

Rycroft C 1972 A critical dictionary of psychoanalysis. Penguin, London

Singer M T, Wynne L C 1965 Thought disorder and family relations in schizophrenics. Archives of General Psychiatry 12: 187–212

Vaughn C, Leff J P 1976 The influence of family and social factors on the course of psychiatric illness. British Journal of Psychiatry 129: 125–37

WHO 1978 International classification of diseases: mental disorders—ninth revision (ICD-9). World Health Organization, Geneva

7

The way to a free and independent life is not to be well cared for. The right way is to train the disabled person to take care of himself.

Battgord

Organisation of rehabilitation services

Clephane Hume

In 1972, the Tunbridge and the Mair reports recommended that a consultant psychiatrist should be appointment to co-ordinate rehabilitation services within each area. The response has been varied. At present, even within one hospital, services may be many and varied. Systems of transitional care do exist, and some have already been described as potential models (Wing and Morris, 1981).

Obviously local needs will dictate requirements, so that one ideal system of care cannot be proposed. But some of the stages that occur in all systems of rehabilitation can be identified. Let us start with the bricks and mortar and consider where rehabilitation programmes may be implemented.

HOSPITAL FACILITIES

The acute admission ward

Acute admission wards may be situated in the psychiaric hospital or district general hospital. They cater for a wide range of newly admitted patients; for some this will be their first hospital admission, but the majority will be readmissions.

Rehabilitation begins with diagnosis (Ch. 2). After the initial assessment, both short- and longer-term goals should be included in the treatment plan. For some patients, only a short stay will be anticipated. Where it is evident that a longer period of rehabilitation is required, referral may be made to a medium-stay ward or rehabilitation unit. Thus, the acute ward staff must be familiar with the referral criteria and treatment approaches used by the other units in order to prepare their patients accordingly.

The contrast between the supportive programme for acutely ill patients and the more demanding schedule for those further on in treatment may cause problems within the acute ward. Acutely ill and disturbed patients require a secure structure which inevitably produces a degree of dependency. To provide, simultaneously, an approach which promotes patient independence and initiative will inevitably create tension. There is a danger that most staff time will be devoted to the care of the acutely ill patients with the less demanding patients being left to look after themselves without the support and encouragement which they need to prevent any deleterious effects of hospitalisation.

The medium-stay ward

Medium-stay wards, where they exist, provide care for patients who require a longer time in hospital before returning to the community. In practice, this will be between one and two years. Most patients will be transferred from an acute admission ward, but some readmissions may be direct from the community when a more prolonged stay in hospital is anticipated.

In the medium-stay ward, the atmosphere will generally be less hectic. Acute symptoms will be under control and there will be more time to consider the practicalities of daily living. Patients will be expected to follow a programme which encourages independence in self-care, self-medication and community integration. Families will be involved in the treatment programme and, if appropriate, a work programme will be initiated.

Most patients will slowly work towards moving out of the medium-stay unit and back into the community. However, a small number of patients will require a further period of support and rehabilitation in a specialised rehabilitation unit or hospital hostel prior to resettlement.

The rehabilitation unit

The rehabilitation assessment unit accepts patients from acute, medium- or long-stay wards and community facilities. This will be the point of entry to half-way houses and hostels where transitional care can be provided. Ideally, it will cater for a small number of patients on a more domestic scale.

Although self-contained accommodation is desirable, the most unlikely wards have been converted into successful rehabilitation units. It is important to provide surroundings which will counteract ward living: small public rooms, bedrooms for, at most, three or four people, kitchen and laundry space, non-institutional furnishings and as many homely details as possible. The need for privacy and personal space must be balanced by the need for some people to experience community living and the social demands and pressures of sharing.

If a range of accommodation can be provided, there is greater scope for individuals to test out their skills in different situations. Any transitional care system should provide the experience of independence available in an unstaffed, but not unsupervised, setting. This enables the patient to be responsible for most aspects of daily living including the implications of having a front door key.

The final placement should provide surroundings in which the patient accepts responsibility for everyday tasks to the maximum extent possible. Ideally, this should be an assessment or pre-discharge flat where furnishings and equipment are on a domestic scale. Patients will be responsible for household management, budgeting their own time, organising social and leisure activities as well as self-medicating from a weekly supply. An allowance for purchasing food and basic necessities may include a budget for heating and lighting. Many patients will have forgotten that lighting, heating and hot water will have to be paid for in the community, unlike the hospital.

If a couple or a group of patients are considering sharing

accommodation, their compatibility may be tested by a period together in a pre-discharge flat.

The long-term ward

Despite being euphemistically labelled as 'rehabilitation wards', long-term wards often provide continuing care or maintenance of chronic patients who have little prospect of ever living outside the hospital. This is often the cinderella of the service in terms of resource allocation, and morale is not improved by the euphemism. False labels lead to false expectations and disappointment. Calling a ward a rehabilitation facility, when it is not, is not helpful to anybody.

Promoting rehabilitation concepts within long-term wards is nevertheless appropriate, although not easy. This requires a change of attitude as much as improved facilities. Steps can be taken to combat institutionalisation by introducing facilities which will promote self-care skills, such as the provision of small-scale tea-making equipment to replace the one-gallon teapots. In addition to personalised clothing and toilet articles, other personal items such as ornaments and photographs are to be encouraged. Domestic staff sometimes object to these because of their dust-gathering potential but this view should be resisted. Tidiness may be sacrified to a certain extent in favour of patient participation. A bed made by the patient may not have the regimented neatness of 'hospital corners', but is much more therapeutic.

Self-medication may be possible within the ward and steps should be taken to simplify administration by initially providing a daily supply. Personal hygiene and care of clothing can be encouraged together with social and communication skills.

Social activities should include outside visits, and pursuits such as swimming combine physical activity with recreation and the use of public transport. Visits to the local pub or betting shop may already be within the routine of individual patients and such normal pastimes should not be forgotten when drawing up social programmes. The use of activities such as reading the daily newspaper can promote the use of verbal skills in conjunction with an awareness of events in the outside world.

Whenever possible, the patient's self-esteem should be

reinforced by recognition of his individual contribution to activities and he should be encouraged to put forward his own ideas and to take part in some ward decision-making processes. Although the aim of the long-stay ward is to maintain the patient at his best level of functioning, some patients may well improve enough over a long period of time to move on to other rehabilitation facilities.

The hostel ward (ward in the community)

There is a group of long-term patients who do not require the degree of care provided by a hospital ward but who are unable to cope with the unstructured environment provided by a group home or lodgings. To meet this need, some hospitals have responded by opening hostel wards based in the community but providing a moderate degree of support and supervision. Most residents have some daytime occupation and the main staff input will be during the evenings and at weekends.

The size and organisation will vary according to the property available and the skills of the residents. There will be encouragement to participate as fully as possible in daily activities and household chores, and this may include making some meals. Residents, even while retaining in-patient status, derive a feeling of satisfaction at having an ordinary address, and may achieve a relatively high level of integration into the local community.

Other hospital resources

In addition to wards, the hospital will provide leisure and recreation facilities and occupation for many patients. A social centre will offer an opportunity to relax as well as practice of social skills. Whether it is buying a cup of tea or participating in organised activities, there is encouragement to develop inter-personal skills.

Most hospitals will have an occupational therapy department and possibly a separate industrial unit. Work assessments can be carried out and the necessary treatment programmes implemented. It should be remembered that a variety of simulated work opportunities exist within the hospital, the potential depending on local policy and the staff available. Perhaps someone could work with hospital porters or gardeners, help with bed-making in the geriatric wards or run a shopping service for those unable to go out.

Although nowadays obtaining a job may be unrealistic for many patients, the value of an occupational routine has been amply demonstrated (Wing & Brown, 1970).

Non-clinical departments

Within the institution, rehabilitation staff may have to explain their approach in order to get their particular requirements met. For example, it will be necessary to explain why un-cooked meals are required in order to allow patients to cook their own food, and the importance of non-institutional clothing and furnishings. The supplies department might well argue that financial considerations restrict what they can provide. However, frequently it is lack of information, imagination or thought that leads to the bulk purchasing of large quantities of chairs of the same style and colour. Identification of this problem should lead to improvement.

The hospital bus driver, shop assistant and other hospital personnel may well be able to provide additional information about our patients. Patients *do* react differently outside the ward or in the community. The message is that your institution may well have more to offer than you have so far discovered.

Day care

Day care provides a bridge to the community, a bridge that permits two-way traffic. The day centre can provide support after discharge from the ward, or may be used as an alternative to hospital admission.

It is necessary to draw a distinction between the day hospital and day centre. Day hospitals offer assessment and treatment with the range of staff normally found within a hospital, nurses, doctors, social workers and occupational therapists. Day centres, which are generally run by local authorities or voluntary organisations, offer occupation and support rather than treatment. They are staffed by occupational therapists, social workers and care assistants rather than medical and nursing staff.

The provision of day facilities is very patchy and there is little provision in rural areas. One exception is the mobile day hospital provided by the Herrison Hospital in Dorset. The day hospital staff travel to improvised 'day hospitals' in village and church halls thereby offering a limited service to a widely scattered population. Urban services may operate for five or more days of the week compared with the weekly visit of the mobile day hospital.

Medication and continued care clinics

Many hospitals provide a depot medication clinic staffed by psychiatrists and community psychiatric nurses. These clinics, which are often open into the evening to allow working patients to attend, provide support in addition to the main provision of medication and monitoring responses and side-effects.

Systematic reviews may be carried out and the early detection of problems is possible. For some people, the clinic has a social function in an otherwise lonely existence.

Having examined the hospital-based services, it is now necessary to look at those provided in the community.

COMMUNITY FACILITIES

Frequently, the patient's own home will be the most appropriate place in which to provide treatment and support. Other community resources fall into two groups, those provided by the statutory and the voluntary bodies.

Many readers will be familiar with the daunting array of services with which a patient may become involved. Table 7.1 indicates some of the community facilities available.

The National Health Service

The primary health care team may assume full responsibility for the patient's care or share management with the hospital

Table 7.1 Some U.K. community facilities

National Health Service	Local authority and social services	Voluntary	Central provision
Primary care team	Area teams (social work)	Local mental health associations	Financial assistance (D.H.S.S.)
Day hospitals	Day centres	Day centres and social clubs	Training and employment (M.S.C.)
Hostel wards	Hostels	Hostels, group homes	
Community pscihiatric nursing service	Sheltered workshops	Sheltered workshops	
	Home helps	Voluntary visitors	
	—— Meals on wheels ——		
	Housing departments	Housing associations	
	Sheltered housing	Sheltered housing	
	Support groups	Support/self-help groups	

out-patient department. If this is the case, good communication will be necessary between all those involved in his care. The community psychiatric nurse will usually be part of the hospital team but, in some areas, these nurses are attached to individual practices or health centres.

Social services and social work departments

The Chronic Sick and Disabled Persons Act, 1970 and the Social work (Scotland) Act 1968 and the Mental Health Acts (England & Wales, 1983; Scotland, 1984) require local authorities to provide after-care services for people who are or have been suffering from mental disorder. The nature of after-care services is not described in the acts but it is required that the local authority shall co-operate with relevant health boards and voluntary bodies. The Mental Health Acts also require local authorities to appointment Mental Health Officers to fulfil certain duties in respect of making application for compulsory detention of patients.

The lack of clear guidelines for after-care services means that the extent of local authority provision is very variable. In general, day care is often provided for the mentally handicapped (adult training centres) and the elderly with little provision for psychiatrically disabled adults. Sheltered workshops may be excellent or virtually non-existent. Joint enterprises with voluntary organisations are well-established, but are not always available to the psychiatrically disabled.

The hostels provided for ex-patients tend to have a maximum length of stay of two years. Few authorities provide longer term hostel places. Homes for the elderly (part III in England and Wales, Part IV in Scotland) are often hard pressed to cope with the growing elderly population and are reluctant to accept old people with a psychiatric history. In some areas, the provision is so limited that only emergency admissions are contemplated; no patients will be accepted from psychiatric hospitals.

In addition to the Mental Health Officers, area social work teams will include those with special interest in psychiatric problems and those seconded to the psychiatric hospital service.

Department of Health and Social Security (DHSS)

In addition to unemployment ('dole'), sickness and supplementary benefits, a resettlement grant is available to assist patients to set up home after some years in hospital. These and other financial benefits change frequently, so up-to-date Information is required from the DHSS welfare assistant or social worker.

Local housing authority

This is not perhaps a body guaranteed to arouse much interest, but a very important one nevertheless. Liaison with the housing department will be required when a long stay in hospital is anticipated or discharge planned. Confirmation that a tenancy may be retained or assistance in obtaining accommodation may be required. Housing officers and visitors may alert the pyschiatric services when they are concerned about the mental health of any tenant. Contrary to some opinion, these officers are not employed to assist in the eviction of tenants but rather to ensure that they are living in the community in reasonable conditions.

The Manpower Services Commission

There is a network of employment possibilities under the umbrella of the MSC (Table 7.2).

Table 7.2 Employment possibilities under the Manpower Services Commission

Manpower services commission	
Employment services agency	*Training services agency*
Job Centre	Skillcentre
Disablement resettlement officer (D.R.O.)	Training schemes
Disabled advisor	
Employment rehabilitation centre (E.R.C.)	
Community projects	*Voluntary projects programme*
Funding for employment opportunities	Opportunities for the unemployed

For some patients, a visit to the Job Centre may be all that is required. Others may gain a job with the assistance of the Disablement Resettlement Officer (DRO). The Disabled Advisor will liaise with prospective employers and promote opportunities in the locality.

If a period of assessment is required, the individual can be referred to the Employment Rehabilitation Centre (ERC). This referral may be initiated by the hospital staff while the patient is still an in-patient, or at the individual's own request to Job Centre staff. The 6–12 week assessment gives the individual the opportunity to test his aptitude for a variety of jobs. At the end, recommendations will be made regarding suitable work. If further training is indicated, he may be transferred to one of the courses offered by the Training Services Agency Skill Centres.

Attendance at the ERC may be necessary to gain entry to a sheltered workshop. In some parts of the country, Sheltered Industrial Groups (SIGS) are available to provide the chance for small groups to work together in an ordinary industrial setting. An example of this type of provision can be seen in Southampton (Wing & Morris, 1981). At times of high unemployment, there is an emphasis on retraining and the provision of work experience. Some MSC funded community enterprise programmes have recently started. One example is the Sprout Market Gardening Rehabilitation Project in Edinburgh.

The voluntary sector

The extent and range of services and support offered by voluntary organisations is considerable. It includes the provision of accommodation, social clubs, day centres and sheltered work as well as self-help groups and active parliamentary lobbying to promote the interests of the mentally ill.

Some voluntary groups focus on a particular condition, supporting sufferers and their families, and raising money for research: National Schizophrenia Fellowship, Alzheimer's Association and Huntington's Chorea Association. Others, such as local mental health associations (MHAs) deal with all mental health problems. National bodies such as MIND (the National Association for Mental Health) and SAMH (Scottish

Association for Mental Health) have a broad remit including fostering a response from local communities to their own needs and assisting the development of local services and facilities. They aim to generate understanding of the mental and emotional needs of the individuals and communities, and influence the development of policy and the allocation of resources to ensure a more effective response to the problems of emotional stress and mental illness in the community.

The variety of accommodation provided by the voluntary sector is impressive. The range extends from group homes sponsored and supported by local MHAs to large-scale hostels or cluster schemes where individual bedsits adjoin communal kitchens and the therapeutic community living offered by the Richmond Fellowship. Elsewhere, the voluntary organisations have moved in to fill gaps in the hospital service. Hospital resources are often overstretched and focus on those in greatest need. There is often little day care provision for the 25–55 age group and social clubs and drop-in centres run by community organisations such as University Settlements and local churches have complemented the hospital service. Some of these are open at weekends and provide meals as well as company.

The Cyrenian Community provides accommodation and occupation (including hostels and farms) as does the Rudolph Steiner organisation. The total care facilities they offer may be particularly appropriate for younger disabled patients.

Recent trends in unemployment have led several voluntary organisations to establish projects for the unemployed. These include co-ordination of voluntary work, educational schemes and short-term work projects. Bodies such as the National Council for Voluntary Organisations are working towards strategies for dealing with the needs of the long-term unemployed, including training and job sharing.

Not all voluntary organisations have been welcomed enthusiastically by the professionals. MIND was considered by some to be meddlesome and possibly dangerous. Time has shown that, on the whole, these organisations have been fighting *with* the professionals to improve conditions for the mentally ill. Far from being negative and dangerous, they have drawn attention to some of the dubious practices within the Health Service but, perhaps most of all, they have made the general public more aware of mental health issues. Patients and relatives can benefit from involvement with the voluntary sector and the rehabilitation services should ensure good relationships with these organisations.

SELECTION OF PATIENTS FOR REHABILITATION UNITS

So far, this chapter has concentrated on the range of facilities available to the patient and his relatives, both within the community and in hospital. Having set out the framework, it is now necessary to consider how to select the appropriate patients for active rehabilitation and resettlement. Perhaps the most crucial question is who to admit to the rehabilitation unit.

Many worthwhile rehabilitation projects have foundered through poor selection of patients. The balance of patients is vital: disparate patient groups may have very different needs while a predominance of certain conditions may be disruptive.

If a new unit is being established to meet a local need, consideration will already have been given to the particular groups of patients for whom the facility is required. The rehabilitation team should decide on the types of disabilities they feel most equipped to deal with and then deterime their selection criteria and procedure. This baseline planning, which will almost certainly have to be modified, is a worthwhile exercise in identifying team members' hopes, expectations and philosophies. Among the range of criteria for selection to be considered are:

(1) patient motivation;
(2) mental state;
(3) daytime occupation/routine;
(4) staff/patient expectations for outcome;
(5) needs of the unit.

Patient motivation

Is he prepared to work towards being resettled in the community? Reluctance to leave known surroundings should not necessarily be taken as a sign of poor motivation, as all change is anxiety-provoking. Does he feel a need to to change his present life-style? How would he like to see himself in the future? Can he identify long-term goals?

Mental state

Before embarking on a full rehabilitation programme, the patient should have recovered from the acute phase of his illness. He should be at a stage where medication has been stabilised and he will be able to cope with the stresses of change.

Daytime occupation/routine

Although it is unrealistic to expect many patients to obtain employment in the present economic climate, the ability to follow an organised pattern of occupation demonstrates a willingness and ability to co-operate with further aspects of a treatment programme. Establishing the habit of a purposeful daily routine provides a good grounding for the future.

Needs of the unit

The balance of residents at present in the unit should also be considered. Some patients will progress more slowly or will attain more limited goals than others. The unit should try to keep the balance so that more active patients provide all-round stimulation and encouragement.

Other considerations

It is a good idea to see relatives at this stage in order to assess the emotional climate at home. Is he surrounded by well-meaning but over-protective people? Does he have to 'go it alone'? Is the family emotionally charged (high EE) or emotionally neutral? Excessive support is as problematical as its total lack.

The treatment team must have clear ideas about the goals for any individual and their expectations of progress. This must be clearly communicated to the patient's relatives and to the patient himself.

SELECTION PROCESS AND ADMISSION TO THE REHABILITATION UNIT

Clear criteria for admission will simplify the selection process, both for the rehabilitation staff and for those making referrals. Referral letters or standardised referral forms will provide some information, but more detailed information may be sought from those in close contact with the patient's relatives, friends and treatment staff. The use of a standard form, setting out questions about level of self-care and social and domestic skills, gives some indication of which tasks the patient can be expected to perform.

A preliminary visit will give the patient a chance to see round the unit and meet some of the residents and staff. An informal meeting with two or three members of the team over a cup of tea may be less threatening, and therefore of more value, than a larger and more formal meeting. A formal assessment interview should take place within the rehabilitation unit to allow all team members to discuss the suitability of the applicant. Finally, expectations on both sides must be clarified.

Rejection of a patient may be because the referral is premature, and re-referral should be considered in the future. Where the unit is quite inappropriate for an individual, it may be possible to suggest more suitable alternatives. Certainly, for the benefit of all concerned, the decision not to accept the patient should be accompanied by an explanation of the decision in order to help the patient and the referring team to plan alternatives.

The involvement of other patients or residents in the selection process is worth considering. A meeting between the individual and other residents is standard practice in some units, but totally unacceptable to others.

STAFFING

It is a myth to suppose that rehabilitation means fewer staff. The opposite is in fact the case. The setting up of programmes, working closely alongside patients and liaison with other departments and community agencies, requires time and organisation.

Disabled patients require high levels of staffing to enable work with small groups to be carried out. It is impossible to practise activities such as managing to use transport in the community with anything other than very small groups. If the rehabilitation unit is part of a system of care including group homes, staff must be available to provide support to residents on different sites.

The composition and possible problems of the multi-disciplinary team is described elsewhere (Ch. 9). Rehabilitation demands enthusiastic and committed staff. Interested staff should be able to elect to work in rehabilitation rather than the common practice of arbitrarily allocating staff for admin-istrative convenience. In any event, there is a need to en-courage the acquisition and maintenance of therapeutic skills by continuing informal and formal education.

The role of volunteers should be discussed. The value of supportive people, who are not regarded as staff, cannot be underestimated and the placement of community service vol-unteers may offer scope for more extensive involvement. The use of volunteers is not without problems and should be fully discussed before they are introduced.

HAZARDS IN THE UNIT

Potentially hazardous situations are a problem for rehabili-tation staff. If a patient falls off a ladder while learning how to hang curtains, who is responsible for any injuries he may sus-tain? Is it dangerous to let a patient replace a light bulb and what about the Unions? Patients may be in a position of hav-ing to carry out these everyday tasks on their own in the very near future. (Suggestion—get the electrician to teach patients how to tackle such tasks, using equipment which is not switched on.)

The rehabilitation team might find themselves out of step with hospital administration who see clear lines of demar-cation between what staff and patients may do. Again it will be a matter of educating the administration in the objectives and needs of rehabilitation.

PATIENTS

In rehabilitation, the organisation of patients occurs on two levels: the organisation of daily routines and timetables according to the requirements of the unit, and the individual's organisation of his own life within this.

Unless the patient is in a small, self-contained hostel or an assessment flat, he will be subject to the rules and regulations which are necessary for the orderly running of any sizeable community. Conformity may not always be in the best interests of the rehabilitation programme but will be necessary for the good of the group as a whole.

Administrative necessities such as giving out medication at a set time, large-scale meals, tea urns, institutional fitments such as the provision of piped boiling water (Kalamax) and contract supplies are familiar to all but they do not make a positive contribution to independent living. The patient who attended a new day centre at a distance from the parent hospital made a valid point when he said, 'You can tell it's part of the hospital, the chairs are all the same.' And even when attempts are made to use facilities outside the hospital, care must be taken. For example, a local optician provides all hospital patients with identical frames for their spectacles, pink frames for the women, blue frames for the men.

Arranging rotas for dish-washing and table-setting never seems to be as easy as one imagines it ought to be, but shared tasks are part of community life. At the same time, patients require privacy. Providing a bedroom in a quiet part of the unit for a patient working as a nightwatchman may not be easy. Similarly, the early riser may disturb others with his alarm clock and subsequent moving about. (Patients need to be able to get themselves up and most people rely on alarms so it is a good idea to get into the habit.)

Despite these difficulties, it is possible for the individual to organise himself within the institution and he should be encouraged to accept as much personal responsibility as he is able. After he rises, it will be up to him to follow his daily routine unprompted. Staying in bed may mean no breakfast: that is his choice. The routine should be flexible enough to allow a lie-in at weekends. If he is going to be late, it is his responsibility to ask for a meal to be kept for him. As far as possible, he should administer his own medication, should organise his time to fit in shopping around his work routine as well as organising leisure activities. At first the subtle change in emphasis from a ward routine may be stressful, but this will usually improve with time.

The aim is to organise the unit in such a way as to minimise the differences between the unit and the outside world. If possible, budgeting should include having to put aside money for rent, gas and electricity and meals should be cooked by the residents.

A vital part of rehabilitation is helping patients (and staff) to know their own limitations as well as their strengths.

MEETINGS, CO-ORDINATION AND LIAISON

Meetings are the backbone of any psychiatric structure and rehabilitation is no exception. Apart from the usual review or Kardex meetings to discuss progress, review treatment and set further goals, the unit may use a variety of other meetings.

Each meeting should have a clearly defined purpose, time and duration. The range includes administrative or policy making groups, staff sensitivity meetings, community groups to sort out routine administrative problems and rotas, and smaller groups with a fixed task such as pre-discharge or psychotherapy groups.

At longer intervals, other meetings may be indicated: liaison between groups of hospital and community staff to organise future placement for patients and relatives' groups.

The use and abuse of meetings is discussed in Chapter 9.

REFERENCES

Apte R Z 1968 Halfway houses. Occasional papers on social administration No 27. Bell, London
Butterworth C A, Skidmore D 1981 Caring for the mentally ill in the community. Croom Helm, London
Caplan G 1961 An approach to community mental health. Grune and Stratton Inc., New York
Guirguis W, Rayner R, Hurley M 1983 Evolution of planned change in a long stay rehabilitation ward. British Journal of Psychiatry 143: 591–6

Mair A (Chairman) 1972 Medical rehabilitation, the pattern for the future. H.M.S.O., Edinburgh

Olsen R (ed) 1979 The care of the mentally disordered — an examination of the alternatives to hospital care. British Association of Social Workers, Birmingham

Rack P 1982 Race, culture and mental disorder. Tavistock, London

Royal College of Psychiatrists 1980 Psychiatric rehabilitation in the 1980s. Report of the working part on rehabilitation of the social and community psychiatry section. R.C.P., London

Shepherd G 1984 Institutional care and rehabilitation. Longman Applied Psychology, London

Tunbridge Sir R (Chairman) 1972 Rehabilitation. H.M.S.O., London

Wing J K (ed) 1982 Long term community care. Experience in a London borough. Psychiatric medical supplement. Cambridge University Press, Cambridge

Wing J K, Brown G W 1970 Institutionalism and schizophrenia. Cambridge University Press, Cambridge

Praising all alike, is praising none.

*John Gay, **Epistle to a lady***

8

The psychological approach

Jill Birrell and Michael Henderson

Within the field of psychiatric rehabilitation, the psychologist has an important contribution to make towards the assessment and treatment of a wide variety of clinical problems. Usually the major theoretical approach is behavioural in orientation. Behaviour therapy seeks to assess and treat disturbances in behaviour by exploring the learned and environmental causes of abnormal behaviour rather than seeking for underlying unconscious mechanisms.

THE INVESTIGATION AND USE OF ASSESSMENT PROCEDURES

The purpose of assessment is to gather information which will facilitate decision making. It may evaluate the efficiency of a clinical service or the assets and deficits of individual patients. The process of assessment involves collecting data in a systematic manner along chosen dimensions. The information obtained is used to decide whether or not to continue, modify or terminate particular activities. Monitoring is important and reassessment is required at regular intervals.

Assessment of populations such as all long-stay/rehabilitation patients in hospital may be a prerequisite for more specific intervention. For example, information about the number of patients with a given level of disability allows for adequate planning for their needs. It is important in large-scale assessments to gather information about the organisation of the hospital, such as staffing levels and the physical aspects of the ward structure, as well as clinical information about the target population.

A wide variety of techniques is available for the assessment of chronic patients, although the range is less comprehensive than for acute patients. Techniques should be both valid and reliable; that is, they should measure accurately whatever the assessor is trying to assess and should do this in a consistent manner. It may be advantageous to compare the findings with other populations, either patient groups or the general population.

Assessment techniques include the following:

1 Interview techniques

The clinical interview is a commonly used method of assessment. It is effective in exploring the feelings and problems that an individual may be experiencing. The vast majority of interviews are conducted in a loose, unstructured format in which the interviewer determines the types of questions asked. However, if the interviewer is interested in comparing the material gathered with that of another interviewer, there is need to impose structure so that the interviews are comparable. In the structured or standardised interview the interviewer gives questions and prompts in a specific order. Patients are all assessed on the same items in the same manner. Most structured interviews are concerned with the measurement of mental state rather than measuring social and behavioural adjustment.

2 Rating scales

These are the most common forms of assessment for a wide variety of activities in different settings. They rely on observations made over a period of days and are usually completed by nursing staff in hospital or a relative in the home. This is because nurses and relatives or friends have the most contact with patients on a day-to-day basis. The rating scale defines the number and the types of behaviour to be rated in a clear and objective way. The rater is asked to record the degree of ability/disability each patient demonstrates and/or the frequency of the behaviours.

3 Direct observation

These techniques rely on immediate recording of 'target' or chosen behaviours as they occur within a specified time period. While careful categorisation of the behaviours to be noted is a prerequisite for direct observation, no opinion or interpretation of the patient's behaviour at the time of recording is necessary.

Assessment is a skill and assessors must be trained in its methods. Hence, while the staff who have the most contact with a patient on a daily basis are usually in the best position to carry out the assessment, they will need a short and systematic training. However, assessment is not without its drawbacks. Although long-stay rehabilitation patients generally show less fluctuation than acute patients, it is not unusual for a small percentage to show marked fluctuations of mental state and behaviour within a short time period. Such changes may make short-term assessments unrepresentative of a patient's total behaviour. In addition, it may be difficult to assess chronic patients' abilities because of their lack of activity and social withdrawal. It is common to find that behaviour alters in different settings. For example, there may be a difference between a patient's eating behaviour on the ward and in the local coffee shop.

Once the assessment is completed, the results must be communicated to all staff concerned. The assessment results lead to a statement of the shorter and longer term goals for a patient and to a programme of activities to reach the specified goals. The results should be recorded, preferably in a standardised form, in the case notes, the written report being backed up by informal discussion. Reviews should take place regularly and there must be a system to ensure this happens.

Individual psychometric assessments

The psychologist has a unique role to play in the assessment of cognitive or intellectual functioning in individual patients using specific tests. In all cases the first question to be asked is whether or not the assessment is likely to be a useful contribution to an individual's rehabilitation programme. Routine assessment of intellectual functioning is no longer considered appropriate. In certain circumstances however, if one of the aims of an individual's rehabilitation is to seek training or open employment it may be helpful. Using standardised techniques such as the Wechsler Adult Intelligence Scale (WAIS) where age norms are available, the psychologist can attempt to determine firstly, the patient's premorbid or prehospitalisation level of intellectual functioning and secondly, the present level. In this capacity intellectual assessment is part of vocational guidance.

Many assessment instruments are available to detect specific deficits resulting from localised or generalised neurological disorders. These may be the primary disorder suffered by the patient (for example, frontal lobe syndrome) or a secondary disorder (for example, dementia in addition to schizophrenia). The assessment of cognitive function provides valuable information to assist in diagnosis at the time and also to allow comparison following retesting at a later date. Test-retest data give detailed information about a patient's deterioration or progress over specified time periods. This is an important factor to be considered in the rehabilitation programme.

Assessment, if used appropriately, can be of great value in rehabilitation. It allows for informed planning of treatment programmes. A thorough account of a patient's strengths and weaknesses and knowledge of the hospital and/or community resources is the best starting point for a rehabilitation programme.

THE FORMULATION AND APPLICATION OF VARIOUS TREATMENT PROGRAMMES ON A GROUP OR AN INDIVIDUAL BASIS

The techniques described below have been found effective in the treatment of a wide range of maladaptive behaviours that have been resistant to other types of treatment.

Unit based and group rehabilitation programmes

The ward is the basic organisational unit within the hospital for most long-stay and rehabilitation patients. Usually there is some degree of specialisation of function in individual wards with patients of similar abilities and deficits living in the same environment. Such specialisation, where it exists, allows for the establishment of ward-based programmes to modify similar deficits and teach new skills to the patient group as a whole. The most widely known of these programmes is the Token Economy Ward. Social Skills groups are also being increasingly used.

The Token Economy

This is the most researched and frequently cited method of group treatment for chronic psychiatric patients, particularly schizophrenics. The approach stems from the classic work of Ayllon and Azrin (1965) which was later republished as an appendix to their book *The Token Economy* in 1968.

Of primary importance in understanding the approach to therapy are two of the major laws of learning theory; *the law of effect* and *the law of association*.

The law of effect states that the frequency of a behaviour is a result of the effect or consequences resulting from the behaviour. Behaviours that result in a positive effect will be repeated while those that result in a negative effect will decrease in frequency and gradually cease to occur altogether. When a behaviour increases in frequency because of pleasant consequences *positive reinforcement* is said to have oc-

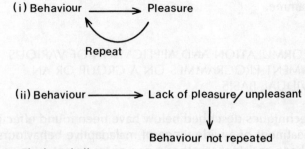

Figure 8.1 The law of effect

curred. When a behaviour decreases in frequency as a result of unpleasant consequences *extinction* has occurred. (See Figure 8.1.)

The law of association states that events which occur closely together in time become associated with one another. Hence a particular behaviour/response becomes linked with the *positive reinforcement* or *punishment* which follows it. At early stages in the learning process the reinforcer must immediately follow the occurrence of the desired behaviour, but at later stages a delay between the occurrence of a behaviour and its consequences is acceptable. In the Token Economy reinforcement is used to change selected existing behaviours. Therapeutic change is brought about by material and social reinforcements administered by staff. Plastic discs or tokens are used as reinforcers in much the same way as money operates in the outside world. In a fully operative token economy almost every behaviour displayed by patients gains or loses tokens. As the staff provide tokens only for desirable behaviours, and withhold them for undesirable behaviours, the patient learns appropriate behaviour. After a stated period of time, the tokens gained can be exchanged for goods or desirable events such as regular time off the ward, privacy, use of the telephone, extra baths, visits to the hairdresser or use of the kitchen. For some patients it can be very difficult to find a suitable reinforcer. Once the behaviour is established tokens can be phased out systematically leaving the individual to show the behaviour as a response to the natural cues of the environment.

Tokens are usually given for the following types of desirable or adaptive behaviour:

(1) Self-care skills: getting out of bed on time, personal hygiene, keeping the bed area tidy, appropriate behaviour at meal times, and so on.
(2) Interpersonal and communication skills: attending and participating in ward activities, responding to requests from members of staff or other patients as appropriate, engaging in conversation and so on.

To be successful the Token Economy requires a vast commitment of time and energy by all members of the multidisciplinary team. The project needs careful organisation prior to its implementation. Consideration must be given to patient assessment and selection, the maintenance of adequate staffing levels both day and night and staff training. Once the programme is running it must be allowed to continue for long enough to produce significant change and vigilance will be required to ensure that the change is maintained. Staff morale cannot be taken for granted and there must be a forum for discussion about any difficulties that arise. If due care is paid to these organisational factors the Token Economy can have longstanding therapeutic effects. The commonest causes of failure are lack of consistency among staff and administrative difficulties. Because most hospitals do not have the resources available to them, only a very small number of Token Economy wards currently exist in the United Kingdom. It is also important to stress that in the absence of a wider supportive network for patients following discharge, a Token Economy is likely to produce no more than temporary and unstable changes.

The social skills training group

Group work may be used to encourage the development of particular sets of skills. A clear example is the Social Skills Training Group. The development of these groups for long-stay/rehabilitation patients is a relatively new departure, although it has long been recognised that social competence is an extremely important factor in successful rehabilitation. Zigler and Philips (1961) found that premorbid social competence of hospitalised psychiatric patients was the best single predictor of post-hospital adjustment.

Social skills (sometimes known as interpersonal or interactive skills) are the skills used in relating effectively to other people. Social skills are pieces of complex behaviour incorporating verbal and nonverbal elements which are necessary for communication with others. Talking clearly and looking at the other person when engaged in conversation is one example of good social skills. Other skills include the use of gesture, appropriate body movements and tone of voice to convey information to others. However, a socially skilled performance involves more than just displaying particular behaviours. It calls for an awareness of the features of human interaction and appropriate responsiveness to what others say and do. Thus the context in which an interaction takes place is important. It would not be appropriate to stand smiling while being told of the death of a relative or friend. Physical appearance in terms of dress, and personal hygiene are also factors to be taken into consideration.

While some social behaviours are innate such as the smiling of a baby, most socially skilled behaviour is learned from observing and modelling upon the behaviour of significant others in childhood and young adulthood. A clear account of the course of 'normal' social development is given by Bandura (1977). While Bandura's approach, known as social learning theory, has its roots in traditional learning theory, it differs quite radically by placing emphasis upon cognition or conscious thought as well as upon direct behavioural phenomena. Also, social learning theory suggests that social skills deficits can be remedied by teaching and training. Indeed, whatever the level of social competence, individuals can be helped to expand their repertoire by a deliberate educational effort, that is, social skills training.

The development of social skills training programmes is due primarily to the work of Michael Argyle, an Oxford social psychologist. The early programmes of the 1960s were developed for college students and shortly afterwards for neurotic outpatient groups, to help them become more assertive and manage interpersonal situations more effectively.

The use of social skills programmes in the area of psychiatric rehabilitation is gaining increasing emphasis. Long-term patients often display a large number of characteristic deficits in social skills. Frequently they are withdrawn, apathetic, uncommunicative and passive in their interaction with others. These behaviours may result from a variety of factors including medication, lack of stimulation in the environment and lack of opportunity for social encounters, in addition to the primary illness. In the initial stages of rehabilitation programmes long-stay patients often have few contacts with people outside the ward and indeed have little need to interact effectively with others as all their basic needs are already met. In moving towards more independent living, however, the ability to communicate one's needs effectively is essential. Hence social skills training should be a vital component of the rehabilitation programme.

1 The assessment of individuals for social skills training

It is important to discover the cause or causes of any social skills deficits. It may be that the individuals have lost social skills as a result of psychiatric illness or that they had never been acquired in the first place. Looking at an individual's premorbid history should help clarify this.

The assessor must also be aware of the patient's current mental state as the presence of psychotic features or high levels of anxiety will make it difficult for a patient to benefit from social skills training. The therapist should consider whether other therapeutic measures, such as chemotherapy for psychotic states or relaxation for anxiety states, are needed prior to or as an adjunct to social skills training. The patient's motivation for participating in a social skills group should also be assessed. Attendance at regular therapy sessions requires a degree of commitment. Individuals need to be motivated to practise newly acquired skills between group sessions by carrying out 'homework' assignments suggested by the therapist.

2 Assessment methods

Assessment methods include the behavioural interview, self report and role play. Investigators have tended to develop new measures rather than improving on existing ones. Most questionnaires and rating scales to date are more applicable to college students and neurotic groups than to long-stay/rehabilitation patients with a history of frequent or long hospital admissions.

It is important to remember that assessment must take account of the particular circumstances of the individual and the facilities available for a training programme. It is insufficient to assess abilities in the hospital ward or hostel alone, for a patient who may be able to chat freely to a fellow patient in such an environment may 'freeze' when trying to engage in similar conversation in the local cafe.

3 Methods of social skills training

Training employs a number of methods which follow each other in sequence (See Figure 8.2). Individuals may be told

Modelling	— demonstrations of ways of coping with particular social interactions
Role play	— group members act out the situations already modelled
Feedback	— comments from observers about the role play
Instructions	— explicit and detailed comments to improve performance
Homework	— tasks set to be accomplished before next formal session
Social Reinforcement	positive feedback from onlookers about an — individual's performance

Figure 8.2 Methods used in social skills training.

and shown how to deal with a specific social situation with which they are finding difficulty. They are then encouraged to practise the situation by role play, followed by the therapist giving feedback to help modify or enhance performance. The situation is then practised again.

An example of a typical social skills programme is given in Figure 8.3. It is important to note that the specific content will vary as a result of the patients' needs and the resources available. The situations practised should be as realistic as possible. Taking the social skills group to a local post office to buy stamps would be more beneficial than only practising in the ward. An initial role play/practice on the ward followed by an outing and a discussion of the trip when back on the ward would be ideal. If the necessary facilities exist it is often helpful to use video and audio recording to allow individuals to watch and listen to their own performance.

The literature on social skills training suggests that individual work is preferable to group work. However, given the demands on the therapists' time group social skills programmes with specific time set aside for individual problems are the commonest format. Usually training groups run for ten to fifteen weeks with six to eight patients in a group and two therapists. It is often the clinical psychologist in the rehabilitation team who is the primary therapist although occupational therapists, nurses and social workers may also be involved as therapists. Frequently the psychologist will act as an advisor rather than an active therapist.

Week 1	— General introduction to the concept of social skills; Body Language
Week 2	— Further body language and vocal expression
Week 3	— Simple greetings, short conversation and leave taking
Week 4	— Longer conversations including self disclosure and complimenting another
Week 5	— Joining and leaving a group; Group conversation
Weeks 6–10	— Continue to practise exercises in Week 1–5. Also coping with criticism, asking for a date, dancing, expressing feelings, assertive behaviour, job interviews

Figure 8.3 A typical social skills programme.

While all staff involved with a patient's rehabilitation programme will not be direct participants in social skills training, each staff member should be aware of the training programme and participate by prompting and praising patients as appropriate. All staff should be issued with a copy of a patient's 'homework' assignments to allow them to give guidance to patients as required.

Individual treatment methods

Assessment of the presenting problem

Psychological intervention begins with the assessment of the presenting problem or problems. A comprehensive history is taken to clarify whether the problem predates hospital admission or has developed in hospital. Careful note is taken of the first occurrence of the problem, any precipitating factors and the consequences of the behaviour for the patient. To complete the history it is usual to record systematically the behaviour of interest or the 'target' behaviour for a specified time. The length of time needed for observation will depend upon the frequency of the 'target' behaviour. The recording may be carried out by the patient in the form of a daily diary. In fact keeping a diary in itself may have a therapeutic effect. It allows the patient to become more aware of the frequency of the behaviour, as well as the events which act as precipitants. The main disadvantage of self-recording is that it may be unreliable. If it seems likely that the patient will not or cannot keep an accurate record, then it is best to employ the services of an outside observer, usually a nurse. However, if the 'target' behaviour occurs outside the ward a relative or other person may act as observer. In either case emphasis is placed upon accurate recording of the time and duration of the 'target' behaviour, and the events that precede and follow its occurrence. An example of a typical recording chart is given in Figure 8.4.

Name			Ward	
Date	Antecedents	Behaviour	Time	Consequences
	Where was the patient? What was happening around him?	What exactly did the patient do and say?	Started/ Ended	What happened as a direct result of the behaviour?

Figure 8.4 The behavioural recording chart.

Treatment methods available

There is a wide range of techniques available for the psychologist to use in individual therapy. These techniques fall into three main headings: (1) The Behavioural Approach; (2) The Cognitive Approach and (3) Other miscellaneous methods.

1 *Behavioural approaches include relaxation, systematic desensitisation, flooding, thought blocking and response prevention.*

Relaxation therapy. Many patients experience excessive tension or anxiety. Relaxation therapy can often help to reduce anxiety. The teaching of progressive muscle relaxation follows a fairly standardised procedure. By alternatively tensing and relaxing different muscle groups the patient learns to discriminate between feelings of tension and relaxation. The first session may take 30 to 40 minutes, after which the patient is instructed to carry out the relaxation exercises on his own. Often a cassette tape of the instructions is given to the patient. The usual minimum amount of time for practice is 30 minutes each day. In the longer term, whenever the patient feels tense or is preparing for a stressful event self-relaxation should be practised.

Systematic desensitisation. This is a technique used mainly for the treatment of phobias. A phobia is an irrational fear of a particular object or situation in the absence of real danger. Some phobias are very specific, such as a fear of spiders or dogs, and some are more diffuse such as a fear of leaving the hospital ward or talking to people. One of the major features of the phobic state is the avoidance of the feared object or setting, and therapy involves reversing this avoidance pattern and encouraging the patient to approach the previously feared situation. A hierarchy of the feared object or situation is drawn up by the patient and therapist. The patient is encouraged firstly to face the least threatening situation and then others in the hierarchy until the most threatening situation is reached. Repeated successful exposure extinguishes the fear reaction and the catastrophe that the patient expected never materialises. Relaxation therapy is an important adjunct to the treatment, allowing the patient to substitute relaxation for anxiety in response to the previously feared object or situation.

Flooding. is another technique used occasionally in the treatment of phobic anxiety states. The patient is not introduced to the feared situation gradually, as in systematic desensitisation, but is asked to spend a long time (up to two hours) in the situation which evokes the most anxiety. Before the first session the patient is given an explanation of what will happen, how long the session will last and how the feeling of anxiety will increase at first and then taper off as the session progresses. It is important to ensure that the patient does not have any means of escape from a treatment session. Relaxation techniques may also be taught to the patient. 'Homework' assignments are given to maintain an individual's exposure to the feared object or situation on a daily basis to supplement formal therapy sessions.

Thought blocking. This is a technique often used to help patients suffering from obsessional thoughts and has also been used in an attempt to reduce the frequency and duration of auditory and visual hallucinations. The patient is asked to engage in the troublesome thought or thoughts and then the therapist interrupts by shouting 'Stop'. The shouting may be accompanied by banging the table or clapping hands. These acts serve to startle the patient and to distract him from the thoughts or hallucinations. The effect of this distraction is pointed out to the patient and then the process is repeated. With frequent practice the patient learns to shout out 'Stop' himself and then to say it silently at appropriate times. An elastic band worn around the wrist and 'pinged' at the same time as saying 'Stop' is another useful and additional distraction exercise.

Response prevention. This technique is used with patients who engage in obsessional rituals such as excessive hand-washing. The patient is introduced to the situation where the obsessional behaviour occurs but is encouraged to stop the indesirable obsessional behaviour before the full ritual is completed. Gradually the patient learns that the full ritual or indeed any of the ritual need not be carried out and that nothing untoward will happen as a result. Thus the patient's anxiety decreases. Sometimes the therapist will model appropriate behaviour in the given situation. The patient may also be taught to relax.

2 The cognitive approach

Cognitive therapy. is a structured, goal-directed, problem-solving approach to the treatment of psychiatric disorders, particularly anxiety states and depression. It is argued that how an individual feels and behaves is a reflection of how he thinks. Negative ideas concerning the person in relation to his environment may have been well rehearsed over a number of years. As with many habits, generally the person is unaware that he is doing this. The principal aims of cognitive therapy are to help the patient recognise his unhelpful negative thoughts, or automatic thoughts, and to replace them with more adaptive cognitive responses.

There are four main stages in cognitive therapy:
 (i) The patient is helped by the therapist to become aware of his negative self-statements and to recognise the relationship between them and changes in mood.
(ii) Having unearthed the maladaptive thought patterns or automatic thoughts, the therapist helps the patient to develop different ways of interpreting events. It is important to remember that the therapist should not impose his ideas on the patient. Instead he should suggest various tasks to enable the patient to discover other possibilities for himself.

(iii) The patient is encouraged to test out his various beliefs and attitudes in a systematic way. The automatic thoughts and the rational alternatives associated with them are regarded as hypotheses the validity of which needs to be determined. Instead of treating ideas as facts, the patient is helped to see that it is possible to discover the truth or otherwise of his beliefs through properly constructed investigations. While the therapy sessions prepare the patient for change, behavioural evidence is required if he is to discard a false belief altogether. One way to bring this about is for the therapist and the patient to design specific assignments which the patient can carry out in the interval between formal therapy sessions.

(iv) As the patient's cognitive style becomes more flexible and clinical improvement is observed, the focus of therapy should move away from the superficial automatic thoughts to the assumptions that underlie them. Unless the latter are identified and modified, the patient is likely to suffer from a recurrence of symptoms at a later date.

There are no strict rules about how many formal therapy sessions are required to complete a course of cognitive therapy. It will depend upon the severity, the amount of patient cooperation and the skills of the therapist. Usually fifteen to twenty sessions over a three month period are sufficient to produce fundamental change. Two sessions per week should be offered in the first month followed by weekly meetings until therapy is terminated. In cognitive therapy, as in behaviour therapy, the treatment hour is overtly structured and the therapist assumes an active role. Generally, a here-and-now locus is maintained. Both schools of therapy endorse the belief that a patient can correct maladaptive behaviour without insight into the precise origins of the problem. Unlike behaviour therapy, however, cognitive therapy seeks not only to produce symptom reduction but to modify attitudes, beliefs and expectations about the self and others.

3 Miscellaneous methods

Biofeedback. The availability of feedback is important in learning how to control internal physiological responses such as heart rate and blood pressure. Since the individual does not receive feedback about these internal events on a day-to-day basis he cannot control them. However, if he is provided with either auditory or visual feedback, he can become aware of the consequences of internal physiological changes and how adjustments can be made to modify and even control them. Blood pressure, heart rate, sweat gland activity, neuromuscular activity and skin temperature can all be controlled by biofeedback techniques.

Although there is a lack of well-controlled studies conclusively demonstrating that biofeedback is an active therapeutic procedure and not merely a powerful placebo, biofeedback has become an important and widely used clinical technique.

General counselling. skills may be used for problems such as social difficulties, unemployment, boredom and difficulties with interpersonal relationships.

Failure to respond to treatment

Sometimes a patient will not or cannot respond to treatment. The failure to respond to treatment should not however be viewed as a complete failure. If the assessment, planning and intervention have been carried out systematically useful data will have been obtained to improve the longer term care of the patient. The patient still requires help to manage difficulties in the long term and the pressures on staff to fall back upon institutional practices must be resisted continually in favour of active, individualised care programmes.

RESEARCH

In addition to the role of the psychologist in assessment and treatment of a variety of clinical problems, he may also be involved in research activities. Belbin (1979) distinguishes between 'applied' and 'applicable' research. 'Applied' research considers major issues of psychological theory such as the theoretical basis of learning. 'Applicable' research on the other hand sets out to solve particular administrative or clinical problems by providing recommendations for their solution. Research carried out within the National Health Service should on the whole be 'applicable' in nature. One example of 'applicable' research has been the development of survey research methods to examine service planning problems. A specific example of this is the work of the Medical Research Council Social Psychiatry Unit on the Camberwell register by Wing and Hailey (1972).

Similar research to produce demographic data about local hospital populations and related services may be worthwhile. Other 'applicable' research might involve the examination of the outcome of various assessment methods and treatments.

There is little to be gained by any profession carrying out research programmes if the results will have no bearing on the work of the rehabilitation team in the care of their patients.

CONCLUSION

The psychologist has a significant role to play in the assessment and treatment of patients with a wide variety of clinical problems. Assessment is the gradual, structured accumulation of information gained from various sources. Accurate assessment is of great value in rehabilitation as it allows for the informed planning of treatment programmes to occur. Treatment involves an intervention which aims to facilitate change towards improvement in patients' functioning. The psychologist has at his disposal a large number of treatment programmes for both groups and individual patients.

In addition to the above skills the psychologist has a role to play in carrying out appropriate research. He also has a contribution to make towards teaching the principles of the psychological approach to other disciplines such as nurses, doctors, occupational therapists and social workers and to liaise with statutory and voluntary agencies outside the hospital to exchange information and advice relating to the rehabilitation unit.

REFERENCES

Ayllon T, Azrin N H 1965 The measurement and reinforcement of behaviour of psychotics. Journal of Experimental Analysis of Behaviour 8: 357–383
Ayllon T, Azrin N H 1968 The token economy. Appleton Century Crofts, New York

Bandura A 1977 Social learning theory. Eaglewood Cliffs, New Jersey
Belbin E 1979 Applicable psychology and some national problems: a synopsis of the 1978 Myers lecture. Bulletin of the British Psychological Society 32: 241–244
Wing J K, Hailey A M 1972 Evaluation of a community psychiatric service: The Camberwell Register. Oxford University Press, London 1964–1971
Zigler E, Philips L 1961 Social competence and outcome in psychiatric disorder. Journal of Abnormal and Social Psychology 63: 264–271

BIBLIOGRAPHY

Beck A T 1976 Cognitive therapy and the emotional disorders. International University Press, New York
Beck A T, Rush A J, Shaw B F, Emery G 1979 Cognitive therapy. John Wiley and Sons, New York
Comrey A L, Bacher T E, Glaser E M 1973 A sourcebook for mental health measures. Human Interaction Research Unit, Los Angeles
Durham R 1983 Longstay psychiatric patients in hospital. In: Shepherd G, Spence S (eds) Developments in social skills training. Academic Press, London
Griffiths R D P 1973 A standardised assessment of the work behaviour of psychiatric patients. British Journal of Psychiatry 123: 403–408
Hall J N 1980 Ward rating scales for longstay patients—a review. Psychological Medicine 10: 277–288
Haynes S N, Wilson C C 1978 Behavioural assessment. Jossey-Bass Publishers, London
Hersen M, Bellack A S 1977 Assessment of social skills. In: Ciminero A R, Calhoun K S, Adams H E (eds) Handbook of behavioural assessment. John Wiley, New York
Hersen M. Bellack A S (eds) 1981 Behavioural assessment—A practical handbook, 2nd edn. Pergamon Press, New York
Honigfeld G, Klett C J 1965 The nurses' observation scale for inpatient evaluation. Journal of Clinical Psychology 21: 65–71
Krowiecka M, Goldberg D, Vaughan M 1977 A standardised psychiatric assessment scale for rating chronic psychiatric patients. Acta Psychiatrica Scandinavica 55: 299–308
Matson J L 1980 Behaviour modification procedures for training chronically institutionalised schizophrenics. In: Hersen M, Eisler R M, Miller P M (eds) Progress in behavour modification. Academic Press, London
Mittler P 1978 The psychological assessment of mental and physical handicap. Harper Row Publishers Inc, United States of America
Van Allan R, Loeber R 1972 Work assessment of psychiatric patients: a critical review of published scales. Canadian Journal of Behavioural Science 4: 101–117
Walsh K W 1980 Neuropsychology. Churchill Livingstone, Edinburgh
Wing J K 1961 A simple and reliable subclassification of chronic schizophrenia. Journal of Mental Science 107: 862–875

We trained hard; but it seemed that every time we were beginning to form up into teams we would be re-organised. I was to learn later in life, that we tend to meet any new situation by re-organising; and a wonderful method it can be for creating the illusion of progress, while producing confusion, inefficiency and demoralisation!

Petronius Arbiter 210 BC

The multi-disciplinary team

Linda Pollock

It is especially appropriate for a nurse to write this chapter. Nurses are central to the functioning of the multi-disciplinary team. They care for patients 24 hours per day and are the culture carriers of the philosophy and treatment programme in a ward. Kushlick (1976), while researching mental handicap settings, established that, on a daily basis, occupational therapists had two to six hours direct contact with patients; doctors and social workers tended to have brief contacts (ten minutes) with more patients in varied situations; but it was nurses who were the key staff of wards, providing 12 hours direct contact.

THE TREND TOWARDS WORKING IN TEAMS

As Hunt (1983) has observed, 'the need to yoke together separate, but interlinked professional skills over the past 20 years has arisen in response to the growth in the complexity of services, the expansion of knowledge and the subsequent increase in specialisations. One person may suffer from limitations of knowledge or experience; a team of different, but inter-related, workers can wipe out these deficiencies.'

As far back as 1959, the *Younghusband Report on Social*

126

Work Services made the point that 'in view of the fast growing complexity and scope of modern knowledge, no one profession dealing with a range of human needs can make exclusive claim in relation to others; each has its essential function as well as its necessary overlap with others. This overlap is required for intelligent cooperation and teamwork. It should also enable an holistic approach to be made to the multiple needs of men.' This sentiment has been endorsed recently by the Royal College of Psychiatrists, who further recommend team work for efficient staff cooperation in the treatment of patients (Royal College of Psychiatrists, 1984).

The benefits of teamwork, then, are that it promotes:
(1) a broader perspective in care provision;
(2) improved communication, leading to:
    (a) shared knowledge and information,
    (b) efficient and optimum patient care;
(3) Consistency of approach and continuity of care.

There is a tendency for the members of a profession to come from similar backgrounds, to have undergone the same sort of training and to hold largely similar views, but these are different from those of other professions. Multi-disciplinary teams thus contain a wider spread of views and experiences than any one profession. Typically, there will be a mix of different ages and professional expertise.

Working as a team encourages better communication between professions. The free interchange of information and views ensures that decisions are made in the light of all the information available. Also, by working closely together, members of different disciplines learn each other's strengths and weaknesses, general professional skills and areas of special interest and expertise. This knowledge can be matched to the treatment tasks to allow the most efficient and effective deployment of staff, with each member concentrating on those aspects with which he is best equipped to deal.

The identification of common goals and objectives at multi-disciplinary meetings ensures that all team members are working to the same plan. This consistency of approach avoids unnecessary confusion to the patient. The availability of team members round the clock provides continuity of care, an informed team member being available at all times. This gives the patient confidence in the staff, and also team members the confidence to 'switch off' when not working, in the knowledge that the patient will not be left unsupported.

REHABILITATION AND TEAMWORK

Teamwork is important in all fields of health care, but especially in rehabilitation. Here the mammoth task of enabling a patient to return to independent living after mental illness cannot possibly be accomplished by one person or one professional group. Multi-faceted problems require a multi-disciplinary approach.

THE TEAM—A DEFINITION

One definition of a team is, 'the coordination of several people in cooperation, to strive for a common aim.' Usually, teams are associated with competition and this suggestion, combined with the use of the word 'strive', hints at some of the problems which can be evident in our attempts to develop a team that works.

Health goals are, in themselves, difficult to define. Furthermore, they vary according to who is offering the definition. The variety of perceptions of health goals and the assortment of pathways to take to reach these goals, are some of the factors which necessitate the use of the multi-disciplinary approach to psychiatric care. These very differences, however, may be divisive and militate against effective team functioning.

The key concepts involved in defining team work then, are: 'co-ordination of several people', 'in co-operation', and 'towards a common aim'. But what exactly is a team?

MEMBERS OF THE REHABILITATION TEAM

Identifying the membership of any multi-disciplinary team is more difficult than it might at first appear. There are hospital teams and community teams, and some people will be members of more than one team. For the purposes of this chapter the teams described are those generally encountered in British practice, although membership will vary according to local custom and availability of staff.

In rehabilitation, teams fall into three groups:

(1) the core team, those who have direct patient contact in the rehabilitation unit;

(2) the extended team, responsible for servicing the organisation in which the core team works;

(3) the community team.

None of the teams should work in isolation. Inevitably there will be overlaps in both the work done and the personnel involved, as the teams are not mutually exclusive. Efficient communication between all groups is essential.

The core team

This usually comprises social worker(s), occupational therapist(s), clinical psychologist(s), and a variety of doctors, nurses, and auxiliaries. This group of people have direct contact with patients and are responsible for the day-to-day organisation of care.

The extended team

This includes many people with responsibility to the whole organisation rather than just to the rehabilitation team. Some, such as the domestic staff and chaplain, will have a considerable amount of contact with patients while others will only rarely be involved. A further layer is provided by the essential staff who have little or no patient contact, but without whom the organisation could not run: administrators, cooks, porters, telephonists, pharmacists and secretaries, to name but a few.

The community team

This team is less cohesive than the core team. It may include hospital-based personnel: doctors and community psychiatric nurses, and those from statutory organisations such as health visitors and local social workers. But quite a different group is involved outside the hospital setting. In hospital nurses are the main workers with the patient. In contrast, outside the hospital, 24-hour vigilance is usually undertaken by a non-professional (family, flatmate, neighbour or friend). In the community everyone coming into a patient's home in some way contributes directly to patient care. When treatment is based in the home, unlike the institution, the patient is the prime focus of attention.

What about the patient himself? Where does he fit in? Is he involved in and considered part of the team? Does he remain on the sidelines? Is he the poor ball being kicked about from player to player? The models used (Ch. 6) often dictate the role in which the patient finds himself.

Here discussion of the multi-disciplinary team will be limited to the professionals involved in provision of direct patient care in hospital, the core team. The issues which will be developed are equally pertinent to the other teams. The same barriers to effective functioning and the same solutions can be applied to extended and community teams.

TEAMWORK AND THE USE OF MODELS

Team members structure their work by the use of models. The four major models and their relevance to rehabilitation are described in Chapter 6. It is worth repeating that many rehabilitation teams do not use one model to the exclusion of the others. Therapists frequently take a more eclectic approach and use plans derived from all models of care.

BARRIERS TO EFFECTIVE TEAM FUNCTIONING

These barriers can be summarised under the following headings:
(1) Organisational
    intraprofessional factors
    leadership issues
(2) Role conflicts
    role confusion
    skills
(3) Gender
(4) Training
(5) Personality and attitudes

Organisational

Structurally the respective professions have profound differences in organisation which affect teamwork.

Intraprofessional factors

Traditionally, nursing is hierarchically organised with beaureaucratic control, where accountability is upwards and growth is discouraged. This organisational means of control tends to inhibit the nurse, discourages initiatives and assures maintenance of the status quo. In psychiatric nursing, men increasingly rise to the top of the management pyramid, which removes them from direct patient contact. Historically, nurses appear to have assumed a 'caring' function carrying out others' prescriptions.

Nursing, then, as it is organised, is not conducive to shared and equal discussion of patient care. Additionally, it is not always clear if the hierarchical authority is clinical, administrative, or both.

In contrast medicine is organised in such a way that doctors are more autonomous in respect of each other's decisions. Promotion does not necessarily take senior doctors away from patient contact. Doctors have a 'curing' philosophy by training which re-enforces the paternal/expert/authoritarian stereotype which pervades medical teaching. Medicine appears to have a less oppressive organisational structure which is more conducive to individual development, enterprise and healthy discussion. Doctors can make independent decisions and as a result they appear, as a group, to be more able to reach a consensus about goals and decisions.

The social worker, occupational therapist and psychologist in the rehabilitation team, like the doctors, tend to have a less inhibited approach to their work. Individuals have more authority to make their own decisions about how to treat patients. This autonomy prepare the way for effecive team discussion.

Other differences in organisation are evident. Different professions work different hours. Nurses tend to work a shift system which necessitates work at night and weekends. Occupational therapists tend to work only from 9–5, Monday to Friday. Doctors and social workers will operate an on-call service which provides emergency cover at night and weekends.

Nurses are responsible for direct patient care, but unlike other professionals, have few additional commitments. The organisation may impose other constraints on the provision of services by individual professions. Financial constraints may mean that an occupational therapist or social worker is shared between several units. Hospital architecture and geographical location may mean that departments are physically far apart.

Effects of differences in organisation

Clearly, organisational factors affect the team's ability to discuss issues relating to patient care. The rationale underpinning the need for ward rounds and team discussions is that collective wisdom is preferable to individual judgements. This only holds true if group processes facilitate discussion. The way different professions are organised tends to impede this. Dynamics within each profession mean that individuals cannot make equal contributions to discussion.

When a multi-disciplinary team agrees what is best for the patient or ward, it can be unclear as to whether a senior member of one discipline can set aside the decision of the team. Has a team decision any real authority when opposed to a hierarchical management authority? This dilemma can have a seriously adverse effect on inter-professional functioning.

The differing philosophies of the professions can influence provision of care. Nurses are at the point where the social organisation for 'cure' converges with the 'care' system. They are obliged to mediate between the two, perhaps with resulting conflict.

Professional differences in organisation affect the availability of each professional for contact with the rehabilitation unit. Nurses are responsible for the day-to-day running of a ward. Other team members usually have other responsibilities and commitments. This could result in the nursing report or morning Kardex being hurried through and not given the time that it deserves, causing frustration and disruption of team discussions. Nurses may feel they are being left to run the unit without support and that doctors are not interested in rehabilitation. A doctor may feel misunderstood by nurses who show their resentment, but do not seem to understand the extent of his other commitments. Social workers may have demands from patients' relatives as well as from the community, which keep them away from the unit. Occupational therapists may be clinical supervisors and run workshops.

Sharing of scarce resources can cause tensions, jealousies and rivalries between units. There is a danger that departments can become isolated, accepting only formal referrals, and become a specialised service.

Leadership issues

To work effectively teams need leadership. The multidisciplinary approach, as a policy, lacks clarity and is open to different interpretations. The appointment of a leader helps to clarify the aims of teamwork. Striving towards a common goal provides a focus for mutual effort and encouragement.

Further, the team leader assumes responsibility for the coordination of the team's activities. Without this, teams lack cohesion and a sense of common purpose.

The leader can also be seen as a figure who provides support and guidance. The leader ensures that there are adequate opportunities to discuss issues relating to teamwork and tries to encourage all team members to attend. Ideally, if there are tensions or problems in the team, the leader assumes responsibility for giving others the chance to solve them. Leaders should be wary of setting up a meeting every time there is a problem. To be effective and productive, meetings must have a specific aim, otherwise they will degenerate into a time-consuming habit.

The leader may also assume responsibility for developing and maintaining a 'unit' culture. Care must be taken that this does not result in the evolution of an exclusive unit which detaches itself from the organisation, and is at the receiving end of antagonism and resentment.

Status of the leader. Who leads? This depends on the unit. Occupational therapist, doctor, psychologist, nurse or social worker? Any one can be leader, depending on the models currently in use. Different models of care lend themselves to different involvement of the contributing professionals. If the predominant model of care is the medical model, then medical input and control will be most influential; a behavioural model requires the psychologist's perspective. Use of a socio-cultural model lends itself to an all-embracing philosophy, emphasising a sharing of knowledge which focuses on social and cultural awareness, in which the social worker is seen as a major force. Use of the psychotherapeutic model would dictate heavy involvement of psychotherapists and those trained in group dynamics. Ideally the leader should be the most senior member of the profession most involved in care provision. The leader is usually nominated by the organisational set-up of the rehabilitation unit: units funded by the social work department are usually led by a social worker. National Health Service Hospitals generally have a medically trained leader.

Style of leadership. A leader of a team should not be autocratic. Where this is the case all information tends to be channelled through the leader, and there is little or no dialogue between team members. This is typical of pyramidal management style, found in nursing management.

Decision-making. Team members should feel confident about acting on their own decisions, knowing that their judgement will be trusted and supported by the leader and other team members. Decisions often may have to be made when the leader is not available for direct consultation. Autocratic leadership tends to be typical of larger teams, where rigid role demarcation and task allocation is evident. This style of communication is not always the fault of the leader: the team may abdicate their decision-making responsibilities and refer all problems to the leader. In rehabilitation, a more flexible style of leadership is preferable as it is more conducive to encouraging discussion and debate.

Ward rounds perhaps exemplify how teams function, and give an insight into styles of leadership. An informal team discussion, with involvement of the majority of the team members, would suggest flexibility. Where the leader sits at the top of a table and is the recipient of most communications, a more authoritation and structured unit would be suggested.

The leader should clarify for all members of the team where independent action is to be encouraged, where joint decisions are to be made, and in the event of differing views, unify the team behind a common decision.

Role conflicts

Role confusion

The advantage of working as a team is that many professions, by virtue of their specialised training, can contribute insights and new perspectives to rehabilitation work. Each profession carries with it an exclusive set of skills. Failure to identify these professional and personal contributions can lead to role confusion which is inefficient and wasteful of training. Initially in any team there will be role ambiguity; the role a person assigns himself, the role the profession assigns for him and the role the other team members assign to him may be in conflict. This role ambiguity must be clarified, otherwise conflicts within the team will develop, and these issues, if unresolved, will form barriers which adversely affect team functioning.

Skills

Delineation of profession-related skills does not do justice to what each individual professional can offer. The concept of 'key worker' (see later) is far more pertinent. The skills which the individual has are not limited to professional training, but develop with experience and further specialisation. Experience gained from working with a variety of patient groups in differing environments and with different approaches to treatment should not be underestimated. Professional training provides merely a foundation on which future work is grounded.

There is a very much larger area where overlap of skills is evident, such as communication skills, expertise in group work or the activities involved in social adjustment. No one individual profession can claim to be the 'expert'.

It is in this grey area of overlap that conflicts can occur. One team member may feel, by virtue of his training, especially skilled to carry out certain tasks. Another team member may disagree. Conversely, a team member may be particularly skilled in dealing with certain problems but be unaware of this. Jealousies and tensions may result from unresolved issues relating to skills: a nurse may resent the doctor 'taking over' as a group leader, or the fact that the doctor is seen as 'wiser' by patients. The occupational therapist may be jealous that he does not have a separate time allocated for reporting his work. The psychologist may resent only being given 'last resort' referrals, or may feel that he has more to contribute than just constructing and administering psychological tests.

Gender

This is an important issue which may affect team functioning. It could however have been included under organisational factors as structurally medicine and nursing are managed by male practitioners although the majority of junior staff are female. This must affect how both medicine and nursing develop, and is equally pertinent to social work but not yet to occupational therapy.

Our judgements of other professionals are affected by gender and sex-role stereotyping. These issues affect team functioning and as such warrant serious discussion. (For a lengthier treatise see Pollock and West, 1984.)

Ward rounds should offer the team a chance to discuss treatment and set goals. Nurses can be actively discouraged from disagreeing with medical colleagues by the nursing officer (usually male). It can be especially difficult for the female nurse to assert herself against her senior's wishes. An additional difficulty, is that a woman might find it hard to assert herself and to develop autonomy. Some of the reasons for this are as follows: first, she is conditioned to be passive and to seek approval, acceptance and guidance to affirm her own value as a person; second, by virtue of her 'other-centredness' (thinking of others first), the female nurse tends to feel guilty about asserting her own desires, and equates 'goodness' with self-sacrifice (Gilligan, 1979). This may mean that in a team situation (which is superimposed on the existing hierarchical structure) the female psychiatric nurse is unable to demand equal 'air time', e.g. the nursing report is often not given the respect that if deserves. Too often it is hurried through, because other members of the team have other commitments. This is a gender-related issue, because the nurse needs considerable assertiveness to voice her perception of the ward, let alone attempt to change the priorities of other professionals. Women can find it hard to disagree with powerful men in the team.

Other effects of gender are worth mentioning here, as they affect teamwork and functioning. A myth exists around the male team members, that of supposedly superior ability to control aggressive behaviour. This undermines the skill and expertise involved in psychiatric nursing, and relegates the male nurse to role of warder. This can cause tension and dis-contentment within the team as men may be seen as con-trollers and the women as carers.

There is another more visible and tangible effect of gender, that of dress. The virtue of wearing a uniform is that it is pro-fessional, that it disguises personality and age differences and establishes mutual behavioural expectations. Women involved in rehabilitation work tend to wear their own clothes. There-fore, the female team member is left with the problem of con-structing a costume which is protective and descriptive of her role. A woman's clothing, compared to a man's, is much more expressive of her personality, her age and her inclinations. Male dress is not so open to interpretation. As a result the young female worker is faced with many more pitfalls than her male counterpart. Whatever the female team member wears, she cannot disguise her sexuality and as such, she is open to sexual comments and prejudice, which undermine her ident-ity as a professional. Within the psychiatric team whatever she does, wears or says, she may always be seen as a woman first.

Other aspects which need to be taken note of, are that fe-males appear to cope with some aspects of teamwork very differently. Perhaps because of inexperience in decision-making, women tend to go for consensus rather than auto-cratic decisions (Dumas, 1975). Men and women also appear to have different views about subjects such as morality which may influence the decisions they make. These qualities in women could be an asset to team functioning, but might be perceived as individual weakness and inability to manage decisively.

Clearly gender affects individuals working in the team, at very many levels.

Training barriers

Team members have a unique contribution to make to the

team because of their specialised training. This can also lead to problems if an individual's ideas about rehabilitation and the contribution he can make are at at odds with the expectations of others. Training tends to mould people's attitudes and influences their approach to patients.

A few examples will illustrate this. Davies (1974) noted that psychiatric nurses have expectations about their involvement in unit decisions that are not shared by doctors or patients. Psychologists trained to implement behaviour modification programmes may find this sabotaged by nurses who disagree with this approach.

Highly trained members of the team can resent working on an equal basis with less trained individuals. This was particularly apparent in the NHS industrial action of 1982 when arguments about pay and conditions reinforced existing staff divisions, resentments and animosities (Illif, 1984). Workers with less training may also resent being told to carry out various activities which they feel are unrealistic.

So staff divisions can arise because of differences in training and orientation. These have to be looked at and worked on if this barrier to team functioning is to be lessened.

Personality barriers

An advantage of the team approach to care is that the constituents combine to give a very mixed group of people. The variety of ages, cultural and social backgrounds and educational achievements, with respectively varied moral stances and values and life experiences, ensures that problems and solutions are seen from several vantage points.

There is a danger that the differing viewpoints lead to subgroups within the team taking rigid positions of opposition where opinions are polarised and discussion and compromise not feasible.

The personalities of the individual professionals can also be an area of derision. Psychiatric nurses have traditionally been custodial and conservative. Noble (1971) demonstrated that these authoritarian attitudes were a major determinant of their approach to patients.

Frank (1974) has commented that the qualities of caring, empathy and genuineness are important elements in psychotherapy. Clare and Thompson (1981) support the contention that theoretical experience and knowledge is irrelevant to outcome, commenting that personalities are the most important influence on the success or failure of treatment. Despite this Storr (1979) believes that therapists should undergo both theoretical and specialised training.

Huntingdon (1981) points out that occupational ideology arises as a function of work relationships and contexts in which people do thier jobs, and not as a result of individual personalities. This would suggest that occupations select or are selected by particular types of personality which will contribute to the specificity of an occupation's ideology.

Clearly the personalities of team members have implications which directly affect patient care.

TEAM BUILDING—REDUCING THE BARRIERS

In spite of all the potential barriers to teamwork, teams do exist and thrive!

However, they do not do so unless concerted efforts are made to prevent and overcome any of the barriers which may have developed. *Teams Are Built, Not Born*. The professionals involved are thrown together (usually not by choice) and have to work together to clarify their common aims and develop a treatment philosophy or culture.

In the following section, some solutions are suggested to help prevent barriers developing and promote effective teamwork. These solutions will be discussed under the following headings:
(1). Organisational
(2). Role conflicts
(3). Gender
(4). Training
(5). Personality and attitudes

Organisational

As illustrated by Menzies (1970), these can be the most difficult to break down. Ideally, each profession acknowledges and accepts the other's limitation and tries to help each achieve maximum potential. Opportunity to air one's frustrations and anger at these organisational barriers can foster feelings of togetherness and serve to make individuals feel cared for and supported. This can go a long way towards developing team cohesiveness, as well as allowing individuals to release bitterness and anger, which are destructive forces in the team.

The nursing hierarchy has a reputation for being oppressive and defensive. This can only change if managers are given the support to be more flexible and if they can trust the lower levels of the hierarchy to be responsible and accountable for their actions. Team meetings should be the forum where issues of accountability, responsibility, support and trust are discussed.

Opportunity for discussion

Individuals should have opportunity to express opinions and be listened to (and heard). Furthermore, the individuals will feel valued if their opinions are included in the decision-making process. If their contributions are valued and used, hopefully polarisation of feelings and animosity will be minimised. Leadership plays an important part in ensuring that meetings take place, and are used constructively. The decision-making process should be shared and be by consensus.

Confidentiality

What are the limits to confidentiality within a team? This can be an extremely difficult area for the team and for patients.

Rehabilitation demands that certain risks must be taken, but in a responsible manner, after discussion and with the full support of the team. Members need to be able to trust one another, to know that professional and ethical standards are maintained and to stand by each other should some crisis occur. Thus confidences cannot be withheld from other team members as the information may be crucial to decision making. But confidential information shared within the team must be treated as strictly confidential and not discussed outside the core team.

Patients may understandably find it impossible to discuss personal problems in front of the team. Often information about patients is gleaned from one-to-one contacts. The individual therapist must make it clear to the patient that this information will be shared with the team. Younger team members may need help to cope with this. Otherwise they may be trapped into keeping secrets, having promised the patient not to tell other team members.

Confidentiality as an issue may well arise in ward rounds, where time should be made available for discussion. These confidentiality issues throw up ethical and moral questions, often of a very complicated nature, which can only be resolved through group discussion.

Respect

Respect is something which must be earned. It is not something that just happens. In time a 'junior' will respect a 'senior' because the latter is seen to be doing a valuable task. One example of this is of a 'senior' sharing demanding patients, not only choosing interesting or dynamic cases. Conversely nurses will not be respected by a doctor if they are seen to be forever in the duty room drinking coffee. Individuals do have to prove their worth in the team, and action speaks far louder than words.

One example which illustrates respect and also generates it, is the use of referral letters. Inter-team referrals are often verbal, casual and off-hand. The simple activity of writing the same information in a letter not only shows respect to the colleague concerned, but clarifies dates and objectives of treatment plans, and can be helpful in planning and assessing. This also stops patients and plans being forgotten as there is a written record of referral. Details of who is doing what, when and why are then readily available.

Role conflicts

Time needs to be made available to allow the team the opportunity to discuss roles to be played, and skills to be used in everyday work. What people have 'on offer' needs to be known, and regular discussion must take place about individual roles in order to minimise misunderstanding and tensions.

This may take place in different settings and is an ongoing process. Individual skills may emerge in ward rounds when discussing patients, in group feedback sessions, at staff meetings where the team philosophy is on the agenda or in sensitivity meetings where staff relationships are the focus. It will only happen if the majority of the team members meet regularly in an atmosphere where all are able to speak freely.

The concept of 'role blurring' is helpful here: it acknowledges that many professions have similar skills. Watts and Bennett (1984) disagree with this and comment that role blurring is undesirable. If one accepts that role blurring is useful in psychiatry, and particularly in rehabilitation, then the necessity for discussion of roles, skills and who does what, becomes paramount.

The key worker

Having accepted that team members have similar and overlapping skills the concept of the 'key worker' is extremely useful. A key worker is allocated to an individual, and this person co-ordinates and organises the care of that particular patient. The profession of that person is largely irrelevant. What is important is that the key worker has the skills, abilities and motivation to help the patient.

The advantage of using the 'key worker' concept is that work is not duplicated and communication and exchange of information is facilitated, as therapy is directed through one person. Key workers appear to feel especially valued as they have clearly defined tasks, and have responsibility for carrying them out. Ideally, all members of the team should be key workers for different patients and each should take a share of 'problem' patients. This latter aspect of the key worker concept serves to increase team cohesiveness, as seniors are seen not to pick and choose their work.

Acquisition of skills

Individuals possess skills and unique abilities which, by example and modelling can be passed on to other members of the team. Discussion of difficult situations or problems can provide the opportunity to learn. This, of course, can only happen if team members are not threatened and are willing to risk admitting failure. Teaching can take place in the day-to-day meetings and ward rounds, but formal teaching sessions can be helpful. These should be multi-disciplinary, with different levels of experience being involved, and with seniors also showing openness and willingness to learn.

The key worker also learns by feedback. Care should be taken that this is done constructively and unjudgmentally. What is most important is that alternative ways of handling situations are discussed. Supervision only works if the therapists feel free to tell the truth about feelings and actions, without fear of reprimand or of being made to feel inferior. This supervision provides monitoring and support.

Allocation of tasks

Allocating tasks can be viewed as a means of organising work, and also as a way to clarify role confusion and ambiguity. Towell (1975) illustrated that, in psychiatric nursing, rigid routines and task allocation were a solution to the problem of control and caring for large numbers of people with minimum resources.

Differences in experience and status are often reflected in different tasks. Those in the position to allocate tasks can control what the other team members are doing, or indeed 'allowed' to do. Those being told what to do may feel that their potential is not being realised and their talents wasted.

At worst, 'task allocation' could reduce the individual's input to the insulting level of a 'task'. The concept of 'key worker' can avoid this as it takes account of the varied aspects of individual team members (age, sex, personality, class etc), and capitalises on other therapeutic resources. Individuals, as a result, will be more appreciative of each other and their contributions.

Gender

The multiplicity of situations, judgements and perceptions affected by gender mean that, ideally, this should be considered at team meetings and teaching sessions. Mere acknowledgment that these exist is a step in the right direction. Each individual's potential (male or female) should be maximised and not inhibited by sexual stereotyping, and this should reduce tensions and increase job satisfaction all round.

Tierney (1983) and many others, have elaborated the many reasons why nursing is controlled by men. It seems that the trend to employ men at management level will only change if nursing is organised differently (with more flexible working hours and the provision of creches).

The value of 'gender' for role modelling, and for marital and group therapy is taken for granted. These assets, in therapy and in team work, should be made explicit and discussed.

Training

There is a danger that, because of their training, different professions use certain models to the exclusion of others. This can cause problems and divisions.

Ideally, this could be minimised if training could be combined. Particularly in psychiatry, nurses, occupational therapists, social workers, pscyhiatrists and psychologists could benefit from a multi-disciplinary approach to teaching for some aspects of their courses. This could lead to mutual understanding and respect of the different roles from the outset.

Professionally prescribed recording systems, kept in different places, can lead to fragmentation and duplication of information. This also perpetuates professional divisions. Problem-orientated records (Weed, 1968) could foster an understanding of differing roles in the team and provide a team record which is orientated towards problem solving and would be particularly relevant in rehabilitation.

Without, as yet, much combined multi-disciplinary training, mutual understanding and respect for different roles and specialities needs to be fostered. Some of the problems arising from separate trainings can be alleviated by teaching within the team. This promotes understanding of different approaches and allows innovations. Particularly in rehabilitation, where problems can be intractable and chronic, this can also increase staff morale and reduce the risk of 'burnout' developing (See later).

Personalities and attitudes

In order to avoid polarisation of opinions and the assumption of rigid stances within the team, all members' opinions and views should be respected. It is important that everyone tries to understand what individuals are suggesting rather than opinions being dismissed outright. There should be a genuine interest expressed in each other's views. Paradoxically, a team should exhibit a balance between agreements and disagreements. Complete agreement all the time suggests that powerful individuals are silencing dissent, while complete disagreement suggests total entrenchment. This balance is called cohesion and this hinges on the team's ability to accomodate disagreement, which is necessary before roles, tasks and goals can be clarified.

BURNOUT

Prophit (1982) has vividly described 'burnout'. She stated: 'Take the analogy of the flame—the flame dances, gives warmth, energy and light, but it eventually gives out when the energy source is depleted, and there is left the inner core—ashen and dead, giving off no warmth, energy or light.' The analogy of the 'spent' match describes a state of physical, emotional and mental exhaustion, which can occur as the result of working with people over long periods of time in situations that are emotionally demanding (Pines, 1980).

Professionals involved in rehabilitation are particularly at risk of developing the 'burnout' syndrome because they are working with a group of people, many of whom are poorly motivated, chronically relapsing and psychosocially disadvantaged.

The main symptoms of burnout are:
— lack of enthusiasm
— reduced availability (for work and discussion)
— avoidance of people (office door shut)
— reduction of time spent with patients
— poor timekeeping
— 'rule-book' mentality (defensive rather than innovative approach)
— resisting change and development
— unhappiness
— feeling that the job is a waste of time
— the professional becomes less caring, more controlling and less feeling. This attitudinal change is graphically illus-

trated by Dusay (1972) using egograms within a transactional analysis framework (Berne, 1972).

One wonders how many readers recognise these symptoms
in their colleagues or themselves?

The degree of burnout has been compared to first, second
and third degree burns, severity of symptoms and prognosis
being affected by the extent of the damage. In the early stages
the syndrome is reversible but, later on, change may be
impossible.

Burnout is not an inevitable consequence of working in rehabilitation, but it is a risk. The team should discuss ways of
re-organising to combat its development in an individual or
the team.

Measures which can be employed to avoid burnout are
listed below:

At work
— ensure a variety of work each day;
— take real breaks away from the place of work;
— encourage responsibility for and control of one's own
   work;
— provide a built-in feedback and support.

Interface
— allow a switching-off time between home and work
— organize relaxation

At home
— do not take work home;
— alternate work and leisure.

Clearly the multi-disciplinary approach to care can provide
an innoculation against 'burnout'. This will offer prestige and
challenge to team members, enhance effective performance
and help foster an atmosphere which will prevent 'burnout'
developing.

WARD NIGHTS OUT!

These are a most enjoyable team activity which can help prevent barriers developing and offer solutions to existing ones.
Nights out can develop and maintain teams!

Ward nights out can provide an opportunity for staff to relax
and get to know each other in a different setting (pub meal,

skittles . . .). In an informal atmosphere staff can obtain information that is an asset to team functioning. Many team conflicts can be better resolved over a pint, or a G and T!

Some people prefer to maintain a totally professional profile where their social preferences and personal life remain anonymous. They will opt out of ward celebrations. This may divide them from the more sociable members. A social core in a ward that forms a clique can discourage healthy discussion and disagreement within its members. It may bring tensions if personal affairs destroy fruitful team functioning.

Personal problems can affect everyone's daily work. If there is a temporary crisis, the team can cope with a member's reduced functioning for a short time. If the crisis is intermittent or chronic, individual counselling may be indicated, preferably by someone outside the team. Some units cope with personal issues which affect team dynamics as team issues in sensitivity meetings, but this is extremely rare.

Nights out, on the whole, are to be recommended. The benefits far outweigh the disadvantages.

CONCLUSION

For clarification and discussion, the barriers to team functioning have been isolated and discussed as discrete entities, but of course, in reality they are much more complicated and intertwining.

Many of the efforts to reduce these barriers have a knock-on effect which enhances the team's work in other ways. The key worker concept encourages the development of skills, and contributes to cohesion. Nights out may provide opportunity for discussion, leading to change of attitudes and different ways of managing situations.

Teams change rapidly. Staff leave and join, patients come and go, and with each adjustment of the constituents, new issues have to be faced. The team is like a kaleidoscope. With every movement, the whole design and emphasis can change and different features take prominence. Each team member must make sure that the individual colours blend to make a pleasing design which holds together for the good of the patient.

REFERENCES

Berne E 1964 Games people play. Penguin, London

Clare A, Thompson S 1981 Let's talk about me: a critical examination of the new psychotherapies. BBC, London

Davies M K 1974 Intra-role conflict and job satisfaction on psychiatric units. Nursing Research 23: 482–488

Dumas R G 1975 Woman power. Appleton Century Crofts, New York

Dusay J M 1972 Egograms and the constancy hypothesis. Transactional Analysis Journal 2, 3:37

Frank J K 1974 Therapeutic components of psychotherapy. A 25 year report of research. Journal of Nervous and Mental Diseases 159: 325–42

Gilligan C 1979 Women's place in man's life cycle. Harvard Educational Review 49: 431–446

Hunt J 1984 in Clark J, Henderson J Community health. Longman Group Ltd, London

Huntingdon J 1981 Social work and general medical practice: collaboration or conflict. George Allen Unwin, London

Iliff S 1984 Marxism today. October:30–35

Kushlick A 1976 Evidence to the committee of enquiry into mental handicap nursing and care. Dawn House, Winchester

Menzies I E P 1970 The functioning of social systems as a defence against anxiety. A report on a study of the nursing service of a general hospital. The Tavistock institute of human relations, London

Noble M A 1971 Organisational structure, ideology and personality in psychiatric nursing. Journal of psychiatric nursing and mental health services 9: 11–17

Pines A 1980 Characteristics of staff burnout. Schiller Park, MT teleprograms

Pollock L C, West E 1984 On being a woman and a psychiatric nurse. Senior Nurse Vol 1, No 17: July 25th:10–13

Prophit P 1982 Burnout—the cost of involvement, of being human in helping professions. Proceedings on nursing research conference. Edinburgh University, Sept 1981

Royal College of Psychiatrists Report 1984 The responsibility of consultants in psychiatry. The Bulletin of the Royal College of Psychiatrists 8: 123–6

Storr A 1979 The art of psychotherapy. Heinemann, London

Tierney A J 1983 Married momen in nursing. Nursing Times September 7th: 30–33

Towell D 1975 Understanding psychiatric nursing. Royal College of Nursing, London

Watts F, Bennet D H 1983 Theory and practice of psychiatric rehabilitation. John Wiley and Sons, London

Weed L 1968 Medical records that guide and teach. New England Journal of Medicine 270: 593–600

Younghusband Report 1959 Report of the working party on social work in social authority health and welfare services. HMSO, London

I am the family face;
Flesh perishes, I live on.

Thomas Hardy Heredity

10

The family and rehabilitation

Clephane Hume

Hospital admission disrupts the normal pattern of living which, for most people, means disruption of family life. As the illness develops and the individual assumes the role and status of 'patient' his family are required to adjust. The stresses experienced by the family members (parents, children, spouse) prior to the patient's admission are followed by the strains of adjustment; reorganising family life to cope without the absent member, to take over his family tasks, and to incorporate regular visits to the hospital into the daily routine. Often the stresses will be severe enough to precipitate emotional disturbance in close relatives. Relatives of schizophrenics admitted to hospital and of psychogeriatric patients attending a day hospital registered a high enough score on the general health questionnaire to be classified as 'cases' (Gilleard et al, 1984). Relatives will be concerned about the patient's progress and their role in treatment, and apprehensive about their ability to cope when the patient returns home. Additional stresses for the families of longer-term patients include coping with the disability and the effort of sustaining family involvement.

In this chapter 'the family' is used synonymously with 'significant others', although the family group discussed is taken to be that of the average UK nuclear family (parents and children living together) rather than the extended family which

149

is typical in other cultures. In many cases the closest and most important people are not related at all. The importance of long-standing close relationships has been recognised by the new mental health legislation (Mental Health Acts, England and Wales 1983, Scotland 1984) where a person living in the same house as the patient for five years or more may be considered 'for the purposes of the Act, to be the closest relative'. In other cases the closest person to the patient may be an old and trusted friend, a partner or workmate or a neighbour, in which case this person would play a significant part in treatment, as if a family member.

PRE-ADMISSION

Many attempts have been made to assess the family's contribution to causing, or at least contributing to the onset of illness. The theories of Laing, Bateson and Wynne and Singer propose that the development of schizophrenia is an inevitable hazard of growing up in certain kinds of family. It is sad that these theories were accepted uncritically long before they were ever tested scientifically. This is dealt with in more detail in Chapter 6.

In the event parents tend to blame themselves for their children's illnesses. Known inherited conditions, such as Huntington's Chorea, will produce additional guilt even though the parents may have been unaware of the risk at the time of conception. The birth of a mentally or physically handicapped baby is a traumatic event which will precipitate grief for the loss of the expected normal baby. Normal grief includes guilt and anger: 'where did we go wrong?', 'what sin have I committed?'. A similar reaction will be experienced, later in life, by parents who blame themselves for their offspring's schizophrenia. Was their parenting at fault, was their love inadequate? Attempts to cope with the guilt and anger may lead to over-protection and excessive exhibitions of affection which may contribute to the stresses of the family member.

A more profitable area of research has been the study of expressed emotion (EE) within the family (See Ch. 6) and attempts to reduce the effect on the patient.

It is easy to be critical of families who appear overprotective and stifling, and to draw the conclusion that this behaviour has contributed to the development of illness. It is necessary to remember that many of the patterns observed may have developed after and as a result of the illness.

Families may tolerate disturbed behaviour for a considerable time before seeking help. Previous experience and cultural background will influence family reactions so that what is seen as being of major significance to one family may be regarded as trivial and not in the least disruptive by another. Some families believe that they should cope by themselves rather than admit to needing help. Others will suffer in silence rather than endure the stigma of being identified as having a psychiatrically sick member. Finally, some families genuinely do not appear to recognise what is happening.

ADMISSION TO HOSPITAL

Hospital admission is a time of change and adjustment for the patient and his family. For the family it will be a time of relief and distress. Admission brings relief from the stresses of looking after and tolerating the illness behaviour and an acknowledgement that the patient needs to be in hospital. At the same time admission may confirm the family's fears about the seriousness of the condition. The wish to keep in touch with the patient through regular visits will mean alteration to the home routine and may well be costly in terms of travelling time, fares or petrol.

Roles may have to change, with the husband taking over some of the tasks formerly undertaken by his wife or vice versa. While the patient may feel relieved that the family can cope in his absence, the taking over of all his roles may leave him feeling redundant and rejected.

In addition to the informal contact with staff while visiting the hospital, the family may be invited to attend formal interviews. These may be to gather information, provide support or to involve them in joint family sessions with the patient.

Good communication is vital. The aims and likely outcome of treatment must be discussed with the family as well as the patient. Unless this is done the team and family may continue to have conflicting ideas. The resulting mixed messages may make it very difficult for the patient to understand the relevance of particular goals.

Peter's ageing mother regularly travelled several miles to visit and would bring a clean change of clothes to exchange. The rehabilitation team felt that Peter was quite able to launder his shirts and underwear although he was not keen to acquire the necessary skills. The charge nurse carefully explained the reasons for Peter taking over the responsibility for his own washing. His mother cheerfully responded that she had arranged for his sister to take over the laundry when she was too frail to manage it herself. Peter, she said, had never done his laundry and never would. With reluctance the team had to agree that this would probably be the case.

For many years Sandy's wife had coped with his episodes of severe depression, his drinking and his eventual dementia. Finally she decided that she could no longer tolerate the situation and told the team that she was not prepared to have him back again. Her feelings of guilt made her unable to tell Sandy this and she continued to collect him for the occasional weekend visit. Unable to understand why the staff were not encouraging him to spend more time at home, Sandy pressed for a discharge date. Despite support and encouragement, his wife refused to take part in any joint interview, and Sandy, very understandably, would not accept the word of anyone other than his wife. This impasse continued for some months until with the passage of time Sandy realised the true situation. The team were able to help him adjust to life as a long-term hospital resident in a relatively independent environment which provided the care and supervision required.

The longer a patient is in hospital, the less likely it is that relatives will continue to visit. Parents die, siblings move away. Nevertheless it is surprising just how many relatives do continue to visit even after as long as thirty years in hospital.

DISCHARGE

It is usual for a patient to return home for short periods prior to discharge, building up from a few hours' visit to overnight and longer stays. This should not be regarded as a test, rather an opportunity for the patient to familiarise himself with life at home. Seeing the visit as a test and being 'on trial' will put additional stresses on the patient and he is less likely to succeed. Also it gives the patient an opportunity to sabotage the visit if he is reluctant to be resettled. If it is merely to familiarise him with life outside hospital, it does not matter whether the visit is a success or not. It remains an opportunity for both the patient and his family to find their feet and adjust to each other with the necessary support.

The patient will find the experience of being a temporary visitor in his own home strange, and possibly uncomfortable. The situation feels artificial and there is a sense of not belonging. If the relatives are over-solicitous the patient may feel smothered and an invalid, and if they are not attentive he may feel ignored. Involvement in routine tasks such as setting the table and washing up may ease the situation.

When the patient is discharged he may find that in his absence, the family have taken over all his roles. If they see him as fragile or at risk of returning to hospital they may be unwilling to relinquish his former tasks. Nevertheless, it is essential that the patient who returns home should be able to resume as much of his previous role as possible. These problems should be anticipated prior to discharge. The family must be allowed to discuss their assessment of the patient, his capabilities and disabilities, with the team and any misapprehensions must be sorted out. They may be fearful that the patient might relapse immediately should they treat him in the wrong way. They may be scared of disagreeing with him for fear of an aggressive outburst. They may ask for advice. The best advice is probably to try to treat the returning family member as normally as possible.

Sarah, who suffered from a paranoid illness, had found it difficult to cope with running the home and caring for two active pre-school children when her husband was away from home on business. While she was in hospital he managed to care for the children without undue trouble. On returning home her first attempt to prepare an evening meal went sadly wrong because bathing the children took longer than usual. Her husband was supportive but did not take over and she was able to save the situation and her own self-esteem by preparing a simple meal in place of the ruined one.

CHRONIC STRESSES

It is easy enough to appreciate that the family of an addict, the parents and children of the newly divorced, and the single person caring for a dementing parent will all be under considerable stress. It is perhaps not so obvious that dealing with difficult behaviour over a long period of time can become a major problem and a lower level of disturbance will be tolerated.

Surveys in the London borough of Camden indicate that tolerance limits, while obviously varying with the individual situation, may have some common features, particularly in relation to the chronically disabled. Socially unacceptable behaviour, such as bizarre actions or sexual misdemeanours, will upset the general public. The lady who talks animatedly to thin air in the coffee shop will attract curious glances and the man who swears and shouts in the street will be avoided. The family may be left to soothe ruffled feelings, or even to placate those people who respond to abnormality with aggression. To share a house with a person whose behaviour is unpredictable or occasionally violent is a perpetual strain. But it is not only aggression and bizarre behaviour which cause problems.

People who habitually rise early (perhaps owing to institutional regimes?) can disrupt sleep for others. Patients may be importuning, demanding cigarettes or money, and many relatives will give in, in order to buy a little peace. Although all patients receive benefits of some kind, they may be reluctant to part with money or contribute towards their keep, placing an additional burden on their relatives.

Living with someone who is anxious, agitated and repeatedly seeking reassurance, is not only emotionally demanding but irritating. Relatives may be distressed by aggressive thoughts, and even acts, directed against the chronically ill or recovering patient. It may be difficult for staff to achieve rapport with a paranoid individual but for his wife, if she is the target of his suspicions, life may be intolerable.

To most people George appeared quite normal, but he had an encapsulated delusional system centred round the belief that his wife was trying to kill him by putting powdered glass in his food. Despite the deteriorating situation at home, his wife could find no-one who would believe her. They could go out for a meal with friends and George would eat quite normally. Eventually George voiced his delusional beliefs to his general practitioner who referred him for psychiatric help.

Having considered the need for contact with relatives or carers throughout the rehabilitation process, it is now necessary to consider the ways in which support can be provided.

SUPPORT FOR THE FAMILY

The multiple needs of relatives cannot be met unless they are known. A single interview, at the hospital, may fail to identify problems as the relatives are unsure of what the team want to hear. A number of contacts, preferably at home, will be needed if a full picture is to be obtained.

The family require:
(1) Information
(2) Empathy
(3) Advice
(4) Help with relationships.

This support may be given individually, as a family, or through attendance at relatives' groups.

Accurate information can go a long way towards relieving stress as ignorance is not bliss and the relatives' fantasies may be much worse than the reality. A clear description of the nature of the illness, the likely prognosis, and implications of the particular diagnosis, may assist relatives and patient to come to terms with the disability. Patients and relatives who understand the treatment procedures and the reasons for their choice are likely to be more co-operative.

The role of the joint interview cannot be overemphasised. The opportunity for discussion in a supportive and controlled setting may allow contentious issues to be discussed for the first time. This is not to say that emotional outbursts will not occur, but rather that such strong feelings can be expressed safely and used therapeutically.

Many families of a psychiatrically disabled patient will feel that they are different and perhaps unique. They find it difficult to believe that other families feel the way they do and this tends to isolate them. Accurate empathy is needed, communicating that someone is able to understand precisely what these experiences are and the effect they have. This is quite different from sympathy or reassurance. Families do not want to be pitied (sympathised with) or to be told that they are coping well when they are patently not (reassurance); what they require is to know that they are not alone and unique and that at least one other person or the team know precisely what they are going through. Sometimes there will be little more that can be offered.

The advice offered should be limited as there are few hard and fast rules. Questions such as, 'Should we tell him to get up in the morning, or just leave him in bed?', are easily answered by referring to what is normal. Of course it is normal for people to remain out of bed during the day, so should the patient. Other questions, such as, 'Sometimes he does what I ask him without any bother, but at other times he shouts at me and throws things about. What should I do, it's difficult to know when he is so unpredictable?' have no clear answer. A solution can only be found through discussion. What have they tried and what has been the outcome? Perhaps, for someone who is disorganised and unpredictable, the only help is for the family to remain consistent and predictable.

It is not unusual to find that parents have conflicting ideas about how to approach the patient. 'His mother is much too soft with him. What he really needs is to get moving and find a good job of work instead of sitting around all day.' 'His father gets so annoyed with Jimmy being at home all the time, but he really isn't able to do much to help himself.' A series of meetings may be required to modify the situation.

Another useful source of support is the relatives' group. It provides an opportunity to share experiences, anxieties and ways of coping, with others in a similar position. Learning that other families are going through the same difficulties can be helpful in itself, but also valuable learning can take place. Staff may act as facilitators, encouraging openness and discussion, and from time to time, may introduce factual information about the illness, and financial and practical assistance. Meetings may be organised specifically for the families of patients attached to a single rehabilitation unit, or open to all families in the locality. In addition, groups may be run by voluntary or self help organisations such as the National Schizophrenia Fellowship. These meetings may have social benefits for relatives who are lone carers.

Voluntary organisations may also provide help in the form of holidays. Where hospital admission is not possible or appropriate, these holidays provide a break for patient and relatives. Sitting services, particularly for people with physical problems, or confusion, are available in some places. Selected and trained volunteers will stay with the patient while the carer goes out.

The activities of local mental health associations are very variable. Although support for the family may not be the prime objective, provsion of social clubs, for example, will provide this indirectly.

Some families sublimate their needs by becoming active in organisations which seek to improve resources for the psychiatrically disabled and research into treatment. This role of joining together with others to fight for a common goal may offer hope and purpose in the face of severe difficulties, thus bringing relief.

ALTERNATIVES TO THE FAMILY

Not all patients have relatives who are willing or able to care for them, or who are in a position to participate in treatment. Sometimes there are significant others, for example friends or workmates who may fill the caring role, and when this is the case, they should be offered the same level of support as relatives.

During the past few years there has been growing awareness of the problem of long-term hospital residents who have no relative or friend through whom to maintain a link with the community. As a result considerable effort has gone into establishing links on a group or individual basis and various befriending schemes are in operation.

The first group of volunteers to become involved were the hospital league of friends. They enable patients to rehearse social skills as they serve them tea in the hospital café, join in social activities or entertain them in their own homes. The appointment of voluntary services organisers (V.S.O.) further encouraged voluntary help. Local mental health associations are the prime source of support to community group homes where they may give practical and financial help in addition to social support, especially to the newly discharged. Fund raising activities, such as a 'nearly new' shop may fund projects which fall between the health and social services or are not considered to be priorities by either.

Volunteers have two kinds of potential in psychiatric aftercare. First, their personal qualities and empathy, their being 'normal', where professional workers are 'special', make them particularly significant figures for people moving out of a 'sick' role. Secondly, there is a flexibility about the deployment of volunteers, so that they may go outside the existing models of health and social services' priorities (Dartington, 1978). Patterns of voluntary help vary from area to area. Dartington describes two different sytems. The V.S.O. in one hospital was able to attract volunteers from the area in which it was situated to work with patients fairly early in their rehabilitation. Those patients who were getting ready to go out were encouraged to be independent—even of volunteers. This paradox, that patients going to live in the community should be weaned off any dependence on volunteers from the community, was partly explained by the fact that the hospital was sited away from its catchment area. In contrast, the V.S.O. in another hospital was looking to adapt the good neighbour idea so that people living near ex-patients in the community could advise the hospital of anything going badly wrong.

Perhaps the main difference between statutory and voluntary services is that the statutory services have to perform certain tasks and because these services are available to all, they are very careful about extending their obligations. Volunteers are free to be choosy and so can afford to be generous. They do not have to be 'fair', in the sense that prescribes the activities of the statutory service. More than that, they are able to give their time and other resources as they feel appropriate. They are therefore able to give support to residents of group homes that would not be possible in other ways. They can set up and run social clubs that do not have to be determinedly therapeutic in aim, they can just be what the people who come to them want them to be. No pressure is put on volunteers about those they work with getting better. So volunteers may be particularly suited to the work in areas in mental health that do not have the reward of dramatic results. Church, or other religious organisations, also offer a bridging support role, with individuals often quietly providing care and attention for many years. Recently, they have begun to open 'centres' which provide company, support and recreation to anyone in need in the community, not focusing on those with psychiatric problems.

Another alternative to family involvement may be through fostering schemes; either temporary 'holiday visit' arrangements or on a more permanent basis through an individual's being adopted into a substitute family. Some local authorities encourage these schemes, in other cases hospital staff may seek out landladies who are willing to open their doors to the disabled. These ventures should not be confused with the larger scale, more commercially run boarding house schemes, which tend not to provide a family atmosphere.

For some people animals help in rehabilitation. Motivation towards rehabilitation may be enhanced if there is a pet to return home to and it has recently been suggested that cat owners may run a lower risk of developing stress related conditions such as ischaemic heart disease. The cat or dog provides a focus of care which helps to diminish the 'patient' role of the disabled person. The emotionally undemanding but warm response of animals' attention makes the owner feel appreciated and needed. Animals are apparently uncritical and therefore not threatening to the recovering patient who may feel that humans are critical of his attempts to cope. For the individual living alone, a pet provides companionship, but can also be the means of establishing contact with others taking the dog for a walk. Tins of catfood top the shopping list in more than one group home!

FAMILY THERAPY

Families may contribute directly to the treatment programme, may receive support from the rehabilitation team or may become the focus of therapy. During the past few years the emphasis has been placed on the treatment of the entire family using group methods. Family therapy may be based on psychodynamic, behavioural or systems theory (the identification of systems and sub-systems used by the family and then modification of their interaction).

As with all forms of treatment, assessment comes first. Interactions within the family, verbal and non-verbal communication, the patterns and systems employed by family members and their inter-relationship are all studied. Specific roles may be identified; for example information giver or receiver, co-operator or saboteur. It may become apparent that members of the family other than the identified patient may be in need of treatment, or that the patient's problems are largely a result of family dynamics.

Assessment thus leads to formulation of the problems, identification of their cause and any factors responsible for their maintenance. Aims of treatment might include improving communication, altering role function or helping the family to solve particular problems.

Adequate training and supervision is required for both family and group work. The use of co-therapists with different levels of experience is a good training situation for the less experienced. In any large group, and some family groups will be very large, it is difficult for one therapist to observe all that is going on. Use of co-therapists is advantageous. If male and female therapists work together it prevents family members of one sex feeling that they are left unsupported. The therapists may take different roles, one tackling a difficult and threatening topic, while the other supports the family. Above all, in the post-mortem discussion after the family session, two therapists should gain a far greater understanding of what has been happening within the family and the progress of their therapy, then either therapist could manage alone.

CRISIS INTERVENTION

Some may be tempted to dismiss this as a fashionable, but rather shallow concept. In fact, crisis theory has its roots in the early studies of bereavement in the 1940s (Lindemann, 1944) and the practice in Querido's work in the 1930s. Many publications have confused the concepts of crisis intervention and emergency psychiatry, implying that the two are synonymous.

A state of 'crisis' is the individual's emotional response to an event or a set of circumstances, not the event itself. Crisis-provoking situations are not necessarily dramatic, and a person might experience crisis after a run of relatively minor events coming close together over a short period of time. Crises have been divided into maturational, those associated with changing roles and responsibilities throughout life, and life crises, which tend to be less predictable and do not happen to everyone.

In a state of crisis, the person or system (family) is more amenable to outside help, is more likely to change and growth might occur. Most crises last for a few weeks before either resolving or at least subsiding for the time being.

Crisis theory suggests that, to be effective, help must be available as early as possible in the state of crisis. A common but mistaken myth of crisis teams is that they are available to rush out at a moment's notice at any time of the day or night. This comes from a misunderstanding of crisis. Crisis lasts for weeks, and to be effective help must be forthcoming at an early stage (days rather than hours). The help should focus on the family rather than an individual patient, the aim being to enhance the decision-making and coping skills of the whole family.

Crisis intervention:
— Is reality-based (what is happening rather than fantasy)
— Is problem-oriented
— Is time-limited (frequent contacts)
— Is family-oriented
— Avoids dependency
— Places emphasis on outside supports

— Uses more than one therapist
— Uses multiple therapies
— Has limited aims.

The emphasis is on what is happening in the 'here and now' and helping the whole family to return to a more stable state. The aims of crisis intervention are limited to returning to the situation before the crisis occured. At that stage, further contracts may be made with fresh aims.

For some families, intensive help at times of crisis is much more productive than prolonged contact with staff when things are more stable. At times of crisis, real changes in coping ability and family interactions can occur. Chronically disabled patients are at risk of being made a scapegoat by their families and blamed for everything that goes wrong. The crisis approach protects the identified patient from such blame by explaining the problem as something that affects the whole family to a lesser or greater extent. Because they are all involved, they all have a part to play in solving the problem. This shift away from treating the patient towards helping the family to work out ways of coping should lead to increased independence for the whole family and less dependence on the professionals. In common with the rest of rehabilitation work, an eclectic approach, using whatever therapies seem most appropriate, is used in order to get the family functioning as quickly as possible.

CONCLUSION

Families, like patients, are very variable. Psychiatric disorder occurring within a family has a major effect in terms of stress, burden, stigma and the adjustment required. Families, like patients, need support and help through this difficult time. Although some families appear to contribute to the patient's relapse (high EE families), staff must be careful not to be judgemental and blame them. Attempts should be made to change the level of expressed emotion or at least to minimise its impact (See Ch. 6.) Where patients require medium or long-term hospital care, families and patients must be encouraged to keep in contact. A patient who is part of a family should not be treated in isolation. The needs of the patient and the family must be considered. For many patients, a family of any sort is better than no family at all.

REFERENCES

Aguilera D, Messick J 1978 Crisis intervention, theory and methodology. 3rd edn C V Mosby Coy, St Louis

Bancroft J 1979 Sex therapy. In: Bloch S (ed) An introduction to the psychotherapies. Oxford University Press, Oxford ch 7, p 146

Bancroft J H J, Greenwood J 1983 Crisis intervention. In: Kendell R, Zealley A (eds) Companion to psychiatric studies, 3rd edn. Churchill Livingstone, Edinburgh, ch 39, p 692

Barker P 1981 Basic family therapy. Grenada, London Bateson G, Jackson D D D, Haley J, Weakland J H 1956 Towards a theory of schizophrenia. Behavioural Science 1: 251–64

Bentovim A, Gorell Barnes G, Cooklin A 1982 Family therapy. For the Institute of Family Therapy, London. Academic Press, London

Caplan G, Killilea M (eds) 1976 Support systems and mutual help. Grune Stratton Inc., New York

Creer C 1978 Social work with patients and their families. In: Wing J K (ed) Schizophrenia: towards a new synthesis. Academic press, London

Dartington T 1978 Volunteers and psychiatric aftercare. MIND in association with the Volunteer Centre, 29 Lower King's Road, Berkhamsted, Herts, HP4 2AB

Fairburn C, Dickerson M, Greenwood J 1983 Sexual problems and their management. Churchill Livingstone, Edinburgh

Gilleard C J, Gilleard E, Whittick J E 1984 Impact of psychogeriatric day hospital care on the patient's family. British Journal of Psychiatry 145: 487–493

Gilleard C J, Belford H, Gledhill K 1984 Emotional distress amongst supporters of the elderly mentally infirm. British Journal of Psychiatry 145: 172–177

Laing R D 1965 The divided self. Penguin Books, Harmondsworth

Lindemann E 1944 Symptomatology and management of acute grief. American Journal of Psychiatry 101: 141–148

Power P W, Dell Orto A E 1980 The role of the family in the rehabilitation of the physically disordered. University Park Press, Baltimore

Querido A 1968 The shaping of community mental health. British Journal of Psychiatry 114: 293–302

Singer M T, Wynne L C 1965 Thought disorder and family relations of schizophrenics. Archives of General Psychiatry 12: 187–212

Vaughn C, Leff J 1976 The influence of family and social factors on the course of psychiatric illness. British Journal of Psychiatry 129: 125–137

Wing J K (ed) 1982 Long term community care. Experiences in a london borough. Psychiatric medical supplement. Cambridge University Press, Cambridge

Wing J K, Olsen R 1979 Community care for the mentally disabled. Oxford University Press, Oxford

Disabled persons have the inherent right to respect for their human dignity. Disabled persons, whatever the origin, nature, and severity of their handicaps and disabilities have the same fundamental rights as their fellow citizens of the same age, which implies first and foremost the right to enjoy a decent life, as normal and full as possible.

United Nations Declaration on the Rights of Disabled Persons, 1975

11

Mental handicap

Sheila Youngson

A decade after this Declaration, many mentally handicapped people do not have such rights respected and they remain a disadvantaged and largely ignored group. This situation will not change until the general public is prepared to accept mentally handicapped people living and working in their midst, and until policy makers and planners are prepared to legislate for, and provide, the required community resources and financial backing.

INTRODUCTION

Definitions of rehabilitation frequently emphasise a recovery of fitness or health or a reinstatement of former privileges and rights. Since mentally handicapped people can never be 'cured' of their handicap, rehabilitation for them is more specifically defined as full integration or re-integration into community life, and the maximising of individual potential.

A chapter of this length does not allow consideration of all the ways or means of achieving such rehabilitation nor is it possible to discuss all the problems and difficulties that may arise for every individual. The special problems of the severely and profoundly mentally handicapped and multiply handicapped groups will not be considered.

164

WHAT IS MENTAL HANDICAP?

The label of mental handicap indicates either that the normal intellectual functions of the brain have not fully developed for whatever reason, or that acquired functions have been lost, due to disease or damage occurring during the developmental period.

Causes

In only approximately 50–60 per cent of cases can the cause of the mental handicap be identified. Table 11.1 lists some of the better known causes.

Table 11.1 Some of the better known causes of mental handicap

Cause	Example
Infections — prenatal — postnatal	rubella, syphilis encephalitis, meningitis
Metabolic disorders	phenylketonuria, hypothyroidism
Perinatal complications	anoxia, mechanical injury, cerebral palsy
Postnatal traumas	non-accidental injury
Postnatal brain disease	tuberous sclerosis
Congenital malformation of the brain and/or nervous system	hydrocephaly spina bifida
Chromosome abnormalities	Down's syndrome (mongolism) Turner's syndrome Klinefelter's syndrome

Prevention and treatment

Fortunately these conditions can be prevented, treated or at least detected *in utero* and termination offered. (Table 11.2) Genetic counselling should also be available to all prospective parents with evidence of a genetically transmitted abnormality, or with a positive family history.

Table 11.2 Examples of prevention and treatment

Prevention	innoculation to prevent infection during pregnancy e.g. rubella (German measles) amniocentesis e.g. Down's syndrome (with selective abortion)
Treatment	dietary regime in phenylketonuria

Incidence

It is estimated that the incidence of mental handicap in the general population is about three per cent with approximately 0.3 per cent being severely or profoundly mentally handicapped. The level of mental handicap—borderline, mild, moderate, severe or profound,— is estimated from an individual's performance on one of the generally used IQ (intelligence quotient) tests. Sometimes such a score provides only a very rough idea of the individual's potential, as this can be greatly affected by the learning and training opportunities available. Figure 11.1 shows the distribution of intelligence in the general population and the levels of mental handicap as defined by the American Association on Mental Deficiency (A.A.M.D.) classification.

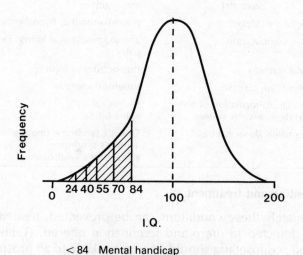

< 84	Mental handicap
70–84	Borderline mental handicap
55–69	Mild mental handicap
40–54	Moderate mental handicap
25–39	Severe mental handicap
< 24	Profound mental handicap

Figure 11.1 The normal distribution of intelligence, showing the cut-off points for the levels of mental handicap, based on the American Association on Mental Handicap classification.
(Not drawn to scale)

HISTORICAL PERSPECTIVE

Before the nineteenth century, mentally handicapped people had at best been tolerated and at worst persecuted. Then pioneering individuals (Jean Itard in Paris, Edouard Seguin in Paris and later in New York, and Samuel Howe in Boston) began to draw attention to the group now known as the mentally handicapped. They showed that, with intensive one-to-one training, individuals previously thought to be incapable of learning even the basics of self-care could in fact be taught many so-called 'higher order' skills such as speech, reading, writing and counting. The establishment of a number of centres to promote such work gave rise to the institutional movement. Numbers of those referred increased and more severely mentally handicapped people were admitted. Progress then halted in the late nineteenth and early twentieth centuries. This was partly a result of the impact of Darwin's theories stressing 'survival of the fittest', and also of the economic depression of the 1930s.

After the depression and with the growth in Britain of the Welfare State, services for the mentally handicapped grew rapidly and various Acts of Parliament began to protect and promote the rights of this group. Perhaps in Britain the most notable was the 1970 Education (Handicapped Children) Act which made it the duty of local education departments to provide education for all handicapped children whatever their level of disability or handicap. Also in the 1970s the philosophy of 'normalisation' came to the fore, stressing that the lives of mentally handicapped people should be as similar as possible to those of the non-handicapped. This philosophy has given impetus to the movement away from hospital care and the growth of alternative community accommodation and training.

It is important, however, to remember that despite the increase in resources and a gradual shifting of attitudes, many myths, prejudices and misconceptions concerning mentally handicapped people still abound. There is a continuing need for public education as doubts, fears and hostility may well adversely affect the setting up and continuation of some community-based projects.

CURRENT PROVISIONS

Institutional care

Traditionally, mentally handicapped people have been cared for in institutions or by their families. Earlier this century (and perhaps as late as the 1960s) many mentally handicapped individuals were admitted to institutions simply because they were mentally handicapped, and not because of any specific needs or problems that could best be dealt with there. It was generally accepted that the care of mentally handicapped people was properly carried out by a hospital service. Many such individuals remain in large, geographically isolated hospitals where little is required of them even in respect of very basic self-care skills.

Institutionalisation

The effects of institutionalisation are far-reaching and are now particularly apparent when many hospitals are trying to relocate their patients in the community. Many patients who may have spent 20 or more years in hospital regard it as their home. (See Ch. 3.)

Any attempt to resettle institutionalised mentally handicapped patients must be a lengthy, time-consuming and gradual process. Sadly it is not always successful. Occasionally, when patients find the move too difficult or stressful, they resort to committing an offence in order to be returned to what they see as a safe and secure environment.

Family care

Increasingly families are caring for their mentally handicapped relative at home. This is partly a result of improved community day-care resources and the reluctance of some institutions to admit patients for long-term care unless there is a need for sustained medical or nursing input.

As in the past, some families keep their handicapped relative at home, devoting their lives to such care.

Overprotection

It is not uncommon to come across elderly parents who have

been looking after their offspring for 40 or more years, without taking holidays, rejecting any social life and effectively isolating themselves and the mentally handicapped person from others. Unfortunately, in these cases, a crisis occurs when illness or death comes to one or both parents. The mentally handicapped person, who has had no experience outside the home and has had all his needs met by his parents, has then to enter an institution as he is incapable of taking care of himself at even the simplest level. The tendency to overprotect the mentally handicapped child is often a problem. This arises particularly when the child reaches puberty and fears about sexual behaviour or sexual exploitation appear. There are many instances of mentally handicapped adolescent girls who are never left unsupervised or are put on the pill 'just in case'. On occasions parents will even ask for their daughter to be sterilised.

Organised support

It would be unfair to suggest that the majority of families fail to cope successfully with their mentally handicapped relative. Many cope well despite mixed and confusing diagnoses, prognoses and lack of organised support. They may spend months and years providing as stimulating and varied an environment as possible, demonstrating apparently endless patience and determination.

The most frequent criticism that families level at services is lack of communication, and this is often justified. What is required is an accessible and well advertised list of available services, agencies and professionals, with a key worker to liaise and coordinate (general practitioner, community nurse, health visitor or social worker).

Family stress

The fact that families of mentally handicapped individuals endure considerable stress for many years must not be ignored. Parental separation or divorce is not uncommon. Often this reflects differing expectations of the mentally handicapped person, differing plans and the restrictions placed on family and social life. Psychological disturbance in siblings may also occur. Many brothers and sisters describe lack of parental attention, frequent requests to help or supervise their handicapped sibling, general family upset and distress and ostracism and teasing from peers.

Little research has been published in Britain evaluating the benefits of parent or sibling support groups but participants often report that such a forum for sharing experiences is of great benefit in putting problems in perspective. As a result, professionals might consider families of mentally handicapped persons as 'handicapped families' and keep in mind the needs and concerns of all those involved.

Education

In most cases in Britain, when a child is of school age, he will attend a local authority school that caters specifically for children with special educational needs. The teacher-to-pupil ratio will be higher than that found in ordinary schools. In some other countries, notably the United States, there has been a movement towards integrating mildly mentally handicapped children into normal classes for as much of the day as possible. However to date this idea has not met with much enthusiasm in Britain.

The curriculum in such schools should include most of the following:

(1) Continued emphasis on *literacy* and *numeracy* skills.
(2) *Self-help skills*: toileting, feeding, washing, dressing.
(3) *Communication skills*: speech comprehension and expression, signing or symbol systems where appropriate, social sight vocabulary (e.g. toilet, exit, stairs).
(4) *Motor co-ordination skills*: running, jumping, throwing, catching, leading to increased body awareness and improved body image.
(5) *Independent living and social skills*: money handling, shopping, travel and traffic, phones, domestic skills, laundry, cooking, personal hygiene.
(6) *Interpersonal relationships*: appropriate and inappropriate behaviours in differing relationships, from casual acquaintance to sexual partner. Sex education and sexual counselling, although many authorities are hesitant to embark on this area.

(7) *Vocational training*: work skills, punctuality, responsibility.
(8) *Leisure activities*: developing interests in hobbies, sports etc.

Until recently, mentally handicapped adolescents left school on attaining the statutory school leaving age. However, since the mid 1970s, it has been increasingly recognised that many mentally handicapped young adults will benefit from continuing school education, perhaps until 18 or 19 years, and some education authorities allow such a provision.

The provision of classes in further education colleges for mentally handicapped people is a promising innovation. This is an increasing though as yet still limited resource. Evening classes, day-release courses and full time courses have been set up for individuals living in institutions or in the community. The content of such courses may include the teaching of skills such as cooking or personal hygiene, literacy and basic education and specific training for employment.

Social service provision: day and residential care

It is the responsibility of regional social service departments in the United Kingdom to provide opportunities to school leavers for further training in a variety of skills and abilities. This usually involves attendance at an Adult Training Centre (ATC) for a number of days each week. The curriculum is likely to include continued basic education, independent living and social skills, art and craft work, physical education and work-related skills. In a very few regions mentally handicapped trainees can graduate through a number of tiers (according to graded ability) and can proceed, where possible, into sheltered or open employment. However, because of the decreasing availability of employment for mentally handicapped people and the long waiting lists for places, many trainees will remain in a particular ATC for many years. It is also the duty of the social services to provide a proportional number of supported accommodation places, usually in hostels. Unfortunately some regions have not met this requirement. In any case this is generally less than the actual need.

Private and voluntary agencies

The deficiency in both day and residential care is fortunately reduced (but by no means eliminated) by the existence of the private and voluntary sector. For example, the Rudolph Steiner organisation provides a range of day and residential care places including sheltered employment. In recent years Housing Associations have also provided accommodation for mentally handicapped people with varying levels of staff support. Some people run 'board and lodging' accommodation catering specifically for mentally handicapped people.

Employment

Despite efforts to encourage the provision of jobs for disabled persons in general, and mentally handicapped people in particular, few realistic opportunities exist. Local authorities in Britain have been slow to build sheltered employment facilities. With the current rise in unemployment, the mentally handicapped group are further disadvantaged. Many of those involved in the care and training of mentally handicapped people think that more emphasis should be placed upon building up leisure and recreational activities, and upon coping with unemployment.

Leisure and recreational activities

This has been a neglected area. Originally emphasis was placed on the label of mental handicap and the provision of separate resources and, latterly, emphasis has been on building up of living skills. What has often been forgotten is the sociability and social needs of the majority of mentally handicapped people. Many voluntary and national organisations have recognised this need and have set up clubs, providing a range of activities for mentally handicapped individuals. These undoubtedly have a place in general rehabilitation and integration. However, the primary objective should be to introduce mentally handicapped people to established community resources, such as sports and community centres and libraries, and to enable them to use and enjoy these resources like other people. Without such an aim there is a danger of setting up mini-institutions in the community with all the usual problems of non-integration and non-acceptance.

FUTURE NEEDS

How can the rehabilitation of mentally handicapped people best be organised to fulfil the definition of rehabilitation?

Assessment of needs

Assessment is not a 'once and for all' definitive evaluation of an individual's current state or future potential. It is a description of that person's skills and abilities, problem areas, and individual difficulties, character and personality and so on, *at that particular time*. This is often forgotten. Assessment should be a regular event, charting progress or deterioration, indicating clearly what has been learned well, what needs further work and what needs encouragement. This is particularly important in the field of mental handicap, when all too often statements are made or scores given that are interpreted as a precise indication of future potential. The IQ score is a common culprit. IQ has often been used as an excuse or justification for individual failure or lack of positive input from professional carers. In fact, much research has shown that an IQ score (whatever it may be measuring) is not always immovable or static, but can change according to the learning, teaching and training opportunities available. The second important consideration under this section concerns the questions:

(1) Why assess?
(2) Who does the assessment?
(3) What should be assessed?

Why assess?

Assessment of an individual may be requested or carried out for a variety of reasons (Table 11.3).

Who assesses?

Who performs the assessment and what is to be assessed will depend on the question or questions to be answered. A wide variety of professions work in the field of mental handicap and each has its own area of speciality (e.g. speech therapy, clini-

Table 11.3 Some reasons for assessment

Investigation of:	Cause for concern:
Specific deficit	e.g. poor speech, or motor co-ordination
Developmental level	e.g. failure to walk or talk at appropriate time
Physical or psychiatric illness	e.g. behavioural change, becoming aggressive or withdrawn
Day or residential requirements (independent living, and social skills)	e.g. ready for discharge from hospital, or no longer able to live at home

cal psychology, physiotherapy and occupational therapy), and its own pool of assessment techniques for particular areas of behaviour (intellectual, developmental, cognitive, social skills, motor skills, verbal and communicative ability, personality, independent living skills etc.). Reports from all members of the team will be required in order to provide a full and detailed profile of the individual, but individual assessments can answer specific queries.

What to assess?

How is the assessment to be carried out? What factors may influence or affect the validity of the results obtained? Assessment can be formal and structured, involving standardised assessment techniques; it can involve questioning and discussion with family, school, social work or nursing staff. It can utilise any mode that provides past or present information, subjective or objective, that will aid understanding, evaluation or prediction of an individual's possible potential.

Problems in assessment

Many factors may affect the accuracy of the final profile. Some of these concern the individual, e.g. his lack of co-operation in the test situation, poor concentration, distractibility or limited communication skills. Some concern the others in his world who may have different standards, perceptions or experiences. The assessor or coordinating assessor must be sensitive and intuitive if a clear and valid assessment is to be obtained.

In an ideal world, as soon as someone is diagnosed as suffering from some degree of mental handicap, the parents or others caring for him should have access to information about all the professions and services available. They need to know how to contact those who can give clarification, support, advice and assistance. Many parents report that they are more or less abandoned for many years after learning of their child's mental handicap.

Better links are required between hospital Paediatric Departments (where the diagnosis is commonly made) and community resources (where support is given). The establishment of Community Mental Handicap Teams in some areas of Britain in recent years is considered to fill this role well. Such teams usually comprise a consultant psychiatrist, a clinical psychologist, nurses, health visitors, social workers, speech therapists, and sometimes occupational therapists and physiotherapists. They offer a community based service to individuals and families, thus also providing a much needed link between the National Health Service and Social Service Departments.

The roles of the National Health Service (NHS) and social services

Currently, in many areas disappointingly poor communication between the NHS and social services exists. This is no doubt partly a result of the much less clear delineation of roles with regard to the care and treatment of mentally handicapped people that now exists. Today, as 'community care' become the watch words and hospitals begin to narrow their admission criteria, social service departments are being asked to provide more resources and personnel. With the present economic climate of financial constraint, debates over responsibility for treatment and care of certain individuals become more frequent.

One solution, in an attempt to avoid such conflict, would be further joint planning of future resources, as well as joint funding of new and innovative community-based projects. At present discussion is under way regarding the possibility of joint training of nursing and social service staff which, should it be implemented, would go some way towards a mutual understanding of work roles and cooperation between services and agencies.

On the other hand, the NHS cannot afford to rest on past laurels. In Britain, despite a policy of moving resources away from acute medicine towards mental health and mental handicap, Health Boards have been slow to act. The NHS must consider what new functions it can best fulfil given the target of increased community care for mentally handicapped people. Over the next 20 years many large institutions will be attempting to reduce their size, and concentrate on caring for the more elderly and more handicapped groups. One other group at least, the very disturbed, will need treatment that perhaps can best be supplied by a NHS resource. The idea of intensive treatment units has been mooted in a number of regions. These could provide treatment for the very disturbed and frequently aggressive patients, perhaps following a behaviour modification approach with a high staff to patient ratio.

Innovations in community care

Assuming that community integration is the aim for most mentally handicapped people, there is a pressing need for more supported accommodation of varying types. Local authority hostels, group homes (flats for a small number of mentally handicapped people with, usually, regular contact with community nurses) and board-and-lodging-type accommodation already exist. These generally provide for the most able, and new concepts in integration should be developed, offering a variety of accommodation and support services for a range of individuals without falling into the trap of creating mini-institutions. Brief mention will be made of two such innovations.

Nimrod

(New Ideas for the Care of Mentally Retarded people in Ordinary Dwellings, a project based in Cardiff) Nimrod aims to provide support, individual training, short-term care and, where necessary, accommodation for all mentally handicapped people in a defined area (in institutions or in the community). By 1983 (four years after inception) the staff team had grown from seven to over 70 (administrative staff, clinical psychologist, social workers, care assistants). Accommodation has been offered to severely mentally handicapped people in 'staffed houses' (24-hour care) and to adults capable of living independently with regular visiting support. The great advantage of such a project is that it identifies *all* mentally handicapped people in a defined area, assesses individual needs, plans individual programmes and monitors progress. It ensures, as far as possible, that each person has the opportunity to maximise his potential, one of the stated aims of rehabilitation. It also crosses professional boundaries and, when good communication is established, provides a unified service to mentally handicapped people living at home or in a residential setting.

The core and cluster concept of housing

This housing concept has been adopted in various parts of the country, and aims to provide ordinary housing for mentally handicapped people living within a defined catchment area. The Core House acts as the administrative base with space for visiting professionals, and as a teaching and training centre. The cluster comprises a number of houses, usually no more than eight, dispersed throughout the defined area thus avoiding the mini-institution label. The houses would be internally designed to cater for a range of needs from minimum support to 24-hour care, and could include single-person, bedsit, co-residence, and staffed accommodation. As with the Nimrod project, once set up, the service could be expanded to provide support, advice and assistance to all mentally handicapped people and families living within the area, including residential assessment and short-term care facilities.

Public education

Any community service or project will only survive and expand if it receives support from local residents. Unfortunately, it is still the case that there is widespread apprehension and even hostility directed towards the mentally handicapped as a group. Much of this is due to the myths and prejudices that exist and are perpetuated through lack of contact with, and understanding of mentally handicapped people.

A public education programme is needed to dispel concerns and fears. Perhaps it would be useful to expand the volunteer worker role within both institution and community in order that familiarity with mentally handicapped people may lead to changes in attitude and perception. Some professionals already visit schools to talk about mental handicap and a beneficial outcome of such meetings is the interest many young people then show in learning more about mentally handicapped people and visiting institutions and day centres.

SPECIAL PROBLEMS

Even if it were widely accepted that mentally handicapped people have the 'right to enjoy a decent life, as normal and full as possible' (United Nations, 1975) it is likely that some difficulties and problems could still act as a barrier towards successful integration or re-integration. Five common problem areas are:
(1) Communication
(2) Behavioural problems
(3) Social skills
(4) Sexuality
(5) Multiple handicaps and psychiatric illness.

Communication

A surprising number of mentally handicapped people have speech and general communication difficulties. This is clearly of paramount importance as it affects all aspects of assessment, treatment and care both from the individual's and the professional's standpoints. Wherever and whenever possible, the mentally handicapped person should be involved in all decision making processes including treatment goals and plans and future placement prospects. Thus he needs to be able to communicate his wishes and needs as clearly as possible. Similarly he needs to understand others' concerns, attitudes, opinions and plans and their implications. The professional involved needs to be able to understand and correctly interpret the messages being relayed. The five areas assessed when a mentally handicapped individual's communicative abilities are being questioned are:

(1) Language comprehension—Does the individual understand what another has said and meant?
(2) Expressive language—Does he successfully communicate his meaning and understanding?
(3) Production of communication—How does he communicate e.g. clear speech, speech approximations, signs?
(4) Additional physical or sensory handicaps—e.g. hearing loss, cleft palate, lack of physical coordination for signing or pointing.
(5) Motivation to communicate—e.g. is he withdrawn or hyperactive, is he easily distracted and lacking in concentration?

Behavioural problems

Lack of adaptive skills

A large number of skills have to be mastered (to some degree) before an individual can live on his own with minimal visiting support. (Table 11.4)

One of the major difficulties encountered is the apparent lack of motivation to change a way of life. The institutionalised adult sitting passively in a chair, the child playing continuously with one favoured toy, are familiar sights. Such behaviour is often the result of earlier lack of learning experience and stimulation which often occur in physically and emotionally deprived environments. The mentally handicapped person, if he is to learn and put such learning into practice, must understand and appreciate the reason why he is being taught a certain skill and have a desired goal for which to aim. For example, the attempt to teach money skills to a hospital patient is unlikely to be successful if he has no opportunity to use money or to go shopping. If he is taken into town, shown desired objects that can be bought and also told that this is a first step towards moving out of the hospital, he is more likely to attend and participate in subsequent sessions.

There are many ways of teaching new skills to mentally handicapped people, and many different settings in which learning can take place. The so-called Behavioural Approach

Table 11.4 The major, basic skills required for independent or semi-independent living

General area	Specific examples
Self-care	eating, toileting, washing, bathing, oral hygiene, dressing and undressing
Use of money	knowledge of coins and notes, handling change, budgeting and saving, Post Office
Shopping	Specialist shops and supermarkets, body size (e.g. waist, chest, hips), shoe size
Domestic skills	hoovering or sweeping, dusting, cleaning rooms, washing, mending, ironing clothes cooking snacks and hot meals, food hygiene, washing dishes
Travel	knowledge of local area, buses and routes, taxis and trains
Safety and health	knowledge of gas, electricity, plumbing, fire and police services What to do and who to contact in an emergency general practitioner, dental services, simple first aid
Literacy and numeracy	social sight vocabulary e.g. ladies, gents, exit, pay here signing name, knowing address, simple addition and subtraction
Concept of time	telling the time, days of the week, date and year
Social behaviour	appropriate basic social exchange, social skills, use of public and private telephone

is often used, providing immediate rewards for acquisition and performance of discrete skills, in conjunction with the identification of longer term goals. Table 11.5 lists some of the strategies that can be used in teaching, along with examples of skills best suited to each strategy.

Maladaptive behaviours

A problem behaviour may be quite difficult to define. A behaviour may be quite acceptable in one setting but not in another (e.g. private versus public masturbation), or the frequency or intensity of the behaviour may determine whether or not it is acceptable. The child who has a mild temper tantrum when thwarted once every three months is not generally regarded as a management problem but if he has prolonged,

Table 11.5 Some strategies that can be used for teaching new skills, and appropriate skill examples

Strategy*	Skill examples*
Shaping	eye contact, using aids, e.g. spectacles, hearing aid, walking frames
Prompting—physical and/or verbal	feeding, washing
Forward chaining	speech, motor co-ordination
Backward chaining	dressing, toileting
Imitation and modelling	teeth brushing, cooking
Graded change	use of feeding, drinking utensils

* Strategies are often used in combination and different strategies can be used for teaching the same skills. Those unfamiliar with the technical terms are referred to Yule and Carr.

violent, screaming temper tantrums twice or more daily, then this is a problem that must be tackled.

Perhaps the closest that can be got to a practical working definition of a problem behaviour is one which poses *a severe physical threat to self or others* (self-injuries or aggressive behaviour), or will lead to that *individual's isolation from others* (e.g. hair pulling, scratching, biting), or will act as *a barrier to future placement* outside a closely supervised and contained environment (e.g. frequent temper tantrums, screaming, verbal abuse, smearing faeces).

With all such problem behaviours the most common treatment approach is a behavioural one. A very detailed analysis is carried out, describing the behaviour in full, the preceeding events and the consequences such behaviour usually brings. The decision has to be made as to where to interrupt this chain of events. Two case histories may illustrate this approach.

John, a three-year-old moderately mentally handicapped boy, had screaming temper tantrums usually two or three times daily. These would occur whenever he wanted a favoured food. His mother would go to him, pick him up, give him cuddles and eventually the food. It was suggested to her that (a) when tantrums occurred she should ignore them as far as was possible, put John in his playpen and leave the room; and (b) when he was behaving well she should give him a lot of attention and physical contact and the favoured food with the words 'Good boy, you haven't screamed, here is a biscuit'. The temper tantrums rapidly decreased, as John learnt that good behaviour meant biscuits, whereas screaming meant no biscuits and the temporary absence of his mother. Therefore the chain was broken by altering the consequences of his behaviour.

Mary, a 45-year-old hospital patient with impaired sight frequently threw crockery and food at meal times. Analysis of this behaviour showed:

(a) that Mary was unable to see her food and was frustrated by not knowing what it was;
(b) that as the dining room noise increased so she became more agitated and ultimately disruptive;
(c) that she sat at a large, particularly noisy table with other disruptive patients who occasionally stole her meal.

It was decided:

(a) to move Mary to a table at the other side of the serving hatch which was much quieter;
(b) to place Mary at a small table with two patients who had good table manners;
(c) to tell Mary what the menu was before she picked up her fork and to guide her hands round the plate so that she knew what was where.

Within a week Mary stopped throwing food and crockery, and indeed her table manners steadily improved. Thus the chain was broken by restructuring her mealtime environment and removing the precipitants of the maladaptive behaviour.

Table 11.6 lists some of the techniques that can be used to decrease maladaptive behaviours. The behavioural approach (also known as behaviour modification, behaviour therapy), is based on a quite complex and involved theoretical framework. (See Yule and Carr, 1980.)

Social skills

Mentally handicapped people often stand out, or fail to be accepted, because of their poor social skills. Often this is the result of impoverished early environments, family over pro-

Table 11.6 Some techniques that can be used to decrease unacceptable behaviours, with examples of such behaviours

Maladaptive behaviour	Technique
Classroom disruption	restructuring the environment
Temper tantrums	extinction
	punishment techniques:
Prolonged aggression	time out from positive reinforcement
Damage to property	response cost/loss of privileges
Self induced vomiting	over-correction
Self injurious behaviour	differential reinforcement of other behaviour (DRO)

tection, general lack of opportunity or lack of correction of mistakes.

Successful rehabilitation or community integration is dependent on mentally handicapped people knowing at least the rudiments of acceptable social exchange and not transgressing the complex and generally unwritten social rules. Assessment in this area often involves no more than taking the opportunity to observe an individual in a variety of social situations and noting where he gets it right or wrong. Sometimes observation *in vivo* is not practical and then techniques such as role play can be used, which are frequently enjoyed by the participants! Individual social skills training and social skills groups have been used, with varying success, in improving social skills. Generalisation of learning is a common problem as is getting across the unwritten rules of social interaction. For example, why is it alright to go up to a stranger and introduce yourself at a disco/dance, but unacceptable in a cafe or restaurant?

Sexuality

A number of mentally handicapped people get into difficulties because of lack of explanation, exploration, understanding and individual acceptance of their own sexuality. All too often they enter and progress through puberty and begin to experience the usual sexual desires and needs with little or no counselling. Frequently this is because of the embarrassment or fears of parents or carers.

Few mentally handicapped people are fortunate enough to be regarded or accepted as sexual beings. It is perhaps not surprising that they sometimes experiment in clandestine ways, and when found out or witnessed, are then labelled as unnatural or perverted.

Unfortunately few visual aids designed for mentally handicapped people are available, an exception being the Winifred Kempton set of slides, entitled *Sexuality and the Mentally Handicapped*. This is a set of over 300 slides (using 'real' people!) covering the whole range of interpersonal relationships, human growth and development, personal hygiene, masturbation, intercourse, contraception, pregnancy and parenthood.

Basic sex education and counselling over the whole gamut of human relationships can be very useful in eliciting the individual's attitudes and perceptions. Various assessment techniques are available, although often professionals have to be quite inventive in order to gain an appreciation of how the individual views himself as a sexual being. This includes attitudes to others as possible sexual partners, and recognising situations as being personal or sexual overtures or openings.

Although there has been relatively little published research on mental handicap and sexuality, it has been shown that, with appropriate sex education and counselling, some mentally handicapped people can embark upon and gain great personal satisfaction from sexual relationships with others. Furthermore they can act in responsible and considerate ways towards their partners. Some have coped well with married life within the community and this includes some mentally handicapped people who have spent many years in institutions. (For further discussion of mental handicap and sexuality, see Craft and Craft.)

Physical handicap, medical problems and psychiatric illness

Some mentally handicapped people have accompanying and often associated physical handicaps. Two common conditions which can lead to such multiple handicaps are cerebral palsy and spina bifida. In such cases the primary task of assessment is to establish learning assets and difficulties so that the environment can be structured to maximise teaching and learning opportunities. Finding and maintaining an efficient, clear channel of communication between patient and professional is of great importance.

Mentally handicapped people are not necessarily more prone to medical or psychiatric illnesses, but neither are they exempt. Some research has shown that they may be more at risk in psychiatric terms than other groups, but it is difficult to separate institutional from individual effects. There are also some medical exceptions to this statement, a notable one being epilepsy which affects approximately 25 per cent of severely mentally handicapped people. A major problem in diagnosis arises when the individual has difficulty in communicating the precise nature of his pain or distress. It is the unfortunate case that occasionally medical or psychiatric conditions will go undiagnosed for a time, any odd or aberrant behaviour being labelled 'difficult' or attention-seeking. A detailed, multi-disciplinary analysis and assessment of the patient, his communications and behaviour, has to be undertaken before a firm diagnosis can be made and a treatment plan can proceed.

REFERENCES

Clarke A M, Clarke A D B (eds) 1974 Mental Deficiency: the changing outlook, 3rd edn. Methuen, London
Craft A, Craft M 1978 Sex and the mentally handicapped. Routledge and Kegan Paul, London
Mittler P 1979 People not patients—problems and policies in mental handicap. Methuen, London
Simon G B (ed) 1980 Modern management of mental handicap—a manual of practice. M T P Press Limited, Lancaster
Yule W, Carr J (eds) 1980 Behaviour modification for the mentally handicapped. Croom Helm, London

Last scene of all,
That ends this strange, eventful history,
Is second childishness and mere oblivion,
Sans teeth, sans eyes, sans taste, sans everything.

William Shakespeare As You Like It

12

The problems
of old age

Ian Pullen

In many societies, one's age is of great importance, both socially and legally. In Britain, it is illegal to leave school, have
sexual intercourse or marry without parental consent before
the age of 16. We may not drive a car before 17 or vote before
the age of 18. Much advertising is aimed at young people who
have a large sales potential and are, therefore, important.

At the other end of the scale, age is also important. In most
occupations, women retire at 60 and men at 65. Officially, as
senior citizens, they are entitled to a State pension and, together with the very young and the handicapped, are exempt
from certain payments. Like the handicapped, they tend to be
treated as a single entity, the elderly.

THE MYTHS OF OLD AGE

The traditional view of old age is spoken by Jaques in the familiar 'Seven Ages of Man' speech quoted above. In other
words, as people get older, their 'minds go'. This is not the
case. Even the very old, those over the age of 80, have only
a one in five chance of suffering from dementia. The vast
majority will retain all their faculties throughout their life, as
witnessed by the University of the Third Age.

Other myths dealt with in this chapter include:
'There are more old people about now because modern medicine is keeping them alive longer;'
'Few people now look after their elderly relations;'
'There is nothing that can be done for the patient with dementia'.
But first, we must consider what happens normally as a person gets older.

NORMAL AGEING

Ageing is a normal biological process that happens to everyone. The rate of progress is very variable and is dictated largely by inherited genetic factors, but may be modified by factors such as trauma or illness.

Physical changes

Many physical changes have been going on slowly for some decades and do not start at the age of 65; however, over that age, change tends to accelerate. Tissues become less elastic, hormone levels change, bones become more fragile and joints show signs of wear and tear. Arteries become less elastic because of atherosclerosis, cardiac output and chest movements are reduced, muscle bulk and strength are lost and the senses decline.

Some of these changes may be masked by plastic surgery ('face lifts') or delayed by diet and exercise (to prevent muscle weakness), but by and large we are powerless to prevent the inevitable decline which has been programmed since conception.

Sexual activity in old age was, for a long time, a taboo subject. Kinsey, in a small sample, found that a fifth of men over 60 were unable to manage sexual intercourse, and that this increased to four-fifths by the age of 80 (Kinsey et al, 1948). Masters and Johnson considered a 'large part of postmenopausal sex drive in women is related directly to sexual habits established earlier in life' (Masters and Johnson, 1970).

Psychological changes

These changes are even more variable than the physical changes. Old people have more difficulty adjusting to new situations and become less likely to change their attitudes. With increased age, memory may be affected. For simple recent memory, this tends to be minimal but may be greater for complex recent memory. The firmly held belief that elderly people have a good memory for long-term events may be illusory. Apparently good recall of past events may arise in part from skilful use of visual memories, and the old person's ability to make detailed statements about past events may be limited to selected topics of emotional significance or topics frequently rehearsed. The problems of measuring intelligence in the elderly are complex as many tests are weighted in favour of younger people. Older people tend to score better on tests which reflect educational attainment (verbal skills) than those measuring performance (coping with new material).

Sociological aspects

Society's attitude to the elderly varies from culture to culture. Traditionally, eastern cultures, where the extended family is the norm, tend to venerate the old, or at least to regard them as important members of the family to be looked after until death. Western cultures have developed a more mobile lifestyle in which the nuclear family and small-scale accommodation more often leave the elderly isolated and alone.

In the West, old age brings retirement with loss of income and status. By contrast, twelve per cent of the oldest men studied in Greece were still working, yet they were more likely than those elsewhere to complain of feeling lonely (WHO, 1983). In Britain, pensions have failed to keep pace with inflation, so that many old people live close to the poverty line. The elderly occupy a disproportionate amount of old and unimproved housing, often having lived there all their married life.

Loneliness, isolation and boredom are common complaints among the elderly. Isolation may result from reduced mobility and may be exacerbated by the death of a spouse and friends, and children moving away. Many feel tired and are poorly motivated to carry on looking after themselves. At the same time, the numbers of the demented and the very frail elderly have meant that an increasing number of the very old are having to live alone, while the more vulnerable are admitted to the often scarce places in local old people's homes and hospitals.

Two main theories set out to describe why old people tend to isolate themselves socially. They are the Disengagement Theory and the Activity Theory.

Disengagement theory (Cumming and Henry, 1961)

This theory suggests that old people cope best if they accept the inevitability of reduced contact with others, particularly the activities of younger people, and manage to enjoy their retreat from the hurly-burly of everyday life.

Activity theory (Maddox, 1963)

Older people, aware of certain failing skills, must make an effort to counteract this deterioration in order to maintain a sense of purpose and satisfaction.

It appears that each theory is correct, but for different groups of old people. Thus, it is necessary to match the old person as each theory suggests a different approach to management. The disengagement theory suggests an acceptance of decline and detachment from the world. Supports should allow the individual to withdraw from social contact and do what he wants. On the other hand the activity theory suggests a more active approach, stimulating the individual to remain sociable, in touch with current affairs and mixing with all age groups (See Reality Orientation below).

Management of normal ageing

The size of the problem: The population of any country depends on the balance between births, deaths, immigration and emigration. In the United Kingdom, since the beginning of this century, births have exceeded deaths, and with the exception of the decades either side of World War II and the late 50s, emigration has exceeded immigration. Not only has the population grown, but the balance of the population has shifted. Since 1900, the numbers of the elderly (aged 65 and over) have increased by over 400%. (Table 12.1)

Table 12.1 Numbers of elderly (in millions) in the UK. (Source: DHSS (1982) Social trends No. 12. HMSO, London. Reproduced by permission)

Year	age: 65–74	75–84	85+
1901	1.3	0.5	
1971	4.7	2.1	0.5
1980	5.2*	2.6	0.6
1991	4.9	2.9*	0.8
2001	4.5	2.8	0.9 (still rising)

* = peak

The total population of the U.S.A. has increased two and a half times since 1900, but the elderly are now six and a half times their 1900 level. This type of change is common to all of the industrialised West.

This is not a result of improved medical care extending the life of very old people.

The life expectancy of a person of 80 today is little different from that the turn of the century. So what has caused the change? In the early decades of this century improved sanitation and food supplies reduced the infant mortality rate. So, quite suddenly, many more children survived childhood. The last two decades have brought further changes. Improved contraception, in particular the Pill, and more permissive abortion legislation have reduced the growth in the birth rate.

So now, in industrialised countries, the elderly account for about 15% of the population compared with a figure of only 3–4% in India and other Eastern countries.

The future

While the 65–74 age group reaches its peak in the early 1980s, the 75–84 age group will peak in Britain in 1991, and the very old, those over 84, will continue to increase into the next century. With advancing age and frailty, old people need more support and practical help with routine day-to-day tasks. The choice lies between maintaining independence with support at home, sheltered housing, or relinquishing independence for the security of an old people's home. The growth in the numbers of the elderly has outstripped the provision of services in many areas, and the situation has deteriorated still further recently because of financial constraints imposed by the Government. While independence is valuable, many old people are being propped up in the community long after this is reasonable because of lack of provision.

Other interventions

Correction of physical and sensory problems is of vital importance. Spectacles or a hearing aid, where required, will make communication easier and may ease the sense of isolation. A community occupational therapist may suggest aids for the home such as large-handled cutlery for weakness of grip. The provision of a trolley to act as a walking frame and to carry things about may make it possible for the old person to move about in safety and without fear. Chiropody and physiotherapy services will add to general fitness. A simple alarm system may remove the fear of being taken ill and of lying unaided for hours or days on end.

Education for retirement and old age

Education should not end because someone is old. Preparation for retirement should anticipate some of the adjustments to be made. Old people must appreciate the need to heat their accommodation adequately during cold weather if they are to minimise the risk of hypothermia. Where possible, open fires should be replaced by gas or electric heaters that are well guarded and fitted with safety mechanisms so that the gas cannot be left on but unignited.

An adequate diet is important and old people must be encouraged to take a varied diet rather than living on jam and tea. They must be informed of the services and benefits to which they are entitled, such as the free incontinence laundry service, and made aware of leisure and social facilities.

Support of the elderly

As an old person becomes slower and more frail, he must rely increasingly on outside support. Often this will be provided by family and friends and the amount of support required varies from person to person.

Informal support

Many old people have a number of people who support them—a neighbour who does some shopping, a grandchild who spends some time with them, a friend who brings in an occasional meal or who takes them out to collect their pension or for a run in the car. Perhaps the regular milkman pauses briefly for a chat and alerts the neighbours if he thinks something is amiss.

This informal support is the most personal, caring, valuable and reliable support that any person can have. It is essential that it is not casually devalued and replaced by temporary professional support. With the best of intentions, home helps, meals on wheels and social work visits can be arranged. If this is carried out thoughtlessly, the informal supporters may suppose that their help was second-rate and amateur and, therefore, retire from the scene. All too soon, the social worker will move on to another area, the home help's days will be cut and the old person decides he cannot afford to contribute to the cost of his meals. By this time, the informal support has evaporated and the old person is less supported than before.

Informal support is the best support and must be encouraged and complemented, not replaced.

Formal support

The provision of services will vary from area to area and it will be a matter or matching services to the old person in question.

ABNORMAL AGEING

Everything so far considered in this chapter relates to the normal process of ageing, not to illness. Abnormal ageing (chronic brain failure or dementia) is a disease process which runs a progressive course over a relatively short period of time, leading ultimately to death. It is quite different from normal ageing.

Although the older a person gets, the higher the likelihood of dementia, only three per cent of those aged 65–70 are demented, rising to only about one-fifth of those over 80. Thus the vast majority of old people, including the very old, are not, and never will become, demented.

Chronic brain failure

Senile dementia is a global deterioration affecting personality, intellect, memory and cognitive functioning. Alzheimer's disease, the most common form of dementia, results in a reduction in the number of nerve cells in the brain and reduced brain size. Less common forms of dementia include arteriosclerotic or multi-infarct dementia, caused by vascular changes to the brain and ensuing damage, and Pick's disease (pre-senile dementia) which affects mainly the frontal and temporal lobes of the brain.

Symptoms of chronic brain failure (See Table 12.2)

Memory: There is a progressive impairment of memory. At first, this is only for recent events, so a shopper may return

Table 12.2 Symptoms of chronic brain failure. (Taken from Isabel Moyes (1980) The psychiatry of old age S,K & F Publications, London, with the permission of the author and the publisher)

personality	intellect	memory	cognitive function
personal neglect	difficulty in abstract thinking	poor short-term memory	poor comprehension
loss of interest and drive	poor reasoning and judgement	poor acquisition of new material	loss of fluency
blunting of emotions	inability to plan ahead	disorientation in time and space	inability to carry out instructions
social misbehaviour	poor concentration		

home without the items he set out to buy. This is largely a deficit of registration rather than of recall, and a simultaneous decline in cognitive function and intellect makes new learning difficult.

The first sign of dementia might be a failure to learn the lay-out of a hotel while on holiday, or inability to locate the toilet when son moves to a new house. Disorientation in place (getting lost) may be followed by disorientation in time (not knowing the time of day, month or year). Later, memory for more distant events is lost and finally memory for self (name).

Cognition and intellect: Poor comprehension and reasoning ability make it difficult to cope with new situations, although regular routines may be unaffected.

Mrs A coped well with shopping daily at the corner shop where she was well known. She bought the same items each day, handing her purse to the shopkeeper who would take out the correct money. She managed by cooking the same meal each day. Then, one day, the local shop changed hands and was turned into a supermarket. Mrs A could not adapt to the change and became confused and frightened. She stopped buying food but, fortunately, this was noticed by a neighbour and a home help was organised. It took only one change to tip the balance with the result that Mrs A failed to cope.

Larger changes, such as a move of house, will have even greater impact.

Poor comprehension may lead to the misinterpretation of events, especially when memory is poor.

An old lady may sit down in a chair placing her handbag at her feet. When she wanders off to another chair, she forgets to take her handbag with her. Looking at her feet, she finds her bag is not where she expects to find it. Mistakenly, she is quite convinced that someone has stolen it.

Although insight may persist for some time with a recognition that memory is impaired, eventually it is lost.

Personality and social functioning

Personality becomes coarsened and self-control and social façade decline. There may be loss of interest and drive, and socially embarrassing situations may arise. Drunkenness, failure to fasten trousers properly, disinhibition, indecent exposure or making sexual suggestions to children may all occur.

Mood is variable and may be blunted or swing rapidly. The frustration threshold may be lowered and the person may use verbal or physical aggression if he has been thwarted. The person's behaviour may endanger others as well, for example, crossing roads without looking or dropping lighted matches or cigarettes.

Physical changes

Most bodily functions are ultimately controlled by the brain. As deterioration proceeds, there may be fits, weight loss, unsteadiness (ataxia) and cardiac arhythmias. Urinary and faecal incontinence reflects a lessened ability to recognise and interpret bodily sensations (as well as difficulty finding the w.c. or inability to walk there quickly enough).

The endpoint, usually after three to five years, is likely to be a chest infection which extends to pneumonia and death.

Management of chronic brain failure

As yet, no specific treatment has been found which will even modify the progress of the dementia, let alone offer any hope of cure. Management must therefore be aimed at minimising handicap and distress, and in common with other forms of rehabilitation, maintaining the best possible level of functioning for as long as possible. The emphasis is on *maintenance* rather than rehabilitation, in the sense of making progress.

Planning

The cornerstone of management is assessment and reassessment. With much of psychiatry, the focus of assessment is the pathology; the abnormal symptoms and signs, the positive family history of illness and disturbance and the problems encountered by the patient. With brain failure, the focus lies not with what is going wrong, but what has been preserved. Of crucial importance is how much healthy function remains.

Where?

Accurate assessment of any elderly patient should begin in his own home. Even a normal old person may perform less competently in strange or intimidating surroundings, such as in hospital. The performance of an old person with impaired comprehension and memory disturbance will deteriorate in strange surroundings. Assessment should be aimed at judging how well a person is able to cope in the familiarity of his own surroundings using his own equipment and local shops. Any assessment away from those surroundings will be of questionable validity.

By whom?

Different members of the clinical team bring different perspectives to the task of assessment, depending on their training and experience (see Ch. 9). The psychiatrist is responsible for making a diagnosis, suggesting any further medical investigations and prescribing medication. The health visitor or community nurse will make a more specific assessment of diet, hygiene and the practical arrangements of daily living including relationships with neighbours and relatives. The occupational therapist is trained to assess the specific skills that are required to live in the community, including cooking, dressing, shopping and cleaning. A social worker may liaise with the family and offer them support and counselling as well as expert advice on financial benefits and local resources that are available.

Of course, these professionals, working as a team, will overlap in their functions. A pattern of working and of individual responsibility is gradually built up so that a fully functioning team does not need to discuss roles.

What to assess?

A general outline is shown below:

(1) *Psychiatric status*

— history
— memory
— reasoning
— misinterpretation — leading to diagnosis
— psychosis
— physical status
— suicide risk
— insight

(2) *Abilities* for daily living
— shopping, cooking, cleaning, organising meals
— managing money, bills, rent
— orientation, house and surroundings
— mobility, public transport, walking
— self-care, washing, clothing, dressing, taking medication
— care of pet, feeding and exercising dog, etc.
— identify any particular dangers.

(3) *Informal support*—Who is doing what, how often, their ability or willingness to do more.

(4) *Formal support*—all those at present professionally involved.

It must then be decided whether any further assessment is required such as specific investigations (CT brain scan, blood tests). After identifying the support that is necessary, the team must determine who can best provide it.

Remember that professional help may be withdrawn at short notice. The informal support of family and friends tends to be more reliable, available at weekends and holiday time; it should never be devalued or replaced without very good reason. The plan should be to fill any gaps with professional help, not to replace the informal support.

Assessment cannot be rushed. The patient must have time to get to know the assessor before attempting any tasks. Even then, the results of the assessment require interpretation according to the individual's circumstances. For example, it does not matter if the patient does not know the day of the week or who is the Prime Minister, as long as she is feeding herself adequately and is generally able to look after herself. In other words, there are no absolutes: it is a matter of weighing up abilities and risks.

Specific supports

The range of support available is shown above (p. 191).

Therapy

The therapeutic work to be carried out with a particular patient suffering from brain failure and his relatives will depend on each individual situation.

Reality Orientation is a basic technique used for people who are disoriented in time, place or person. The aim is to remind people who they are, where they are, the time of day and season of the year, and to keep the person with memory disturbance in touch with the world. Two methods have been investigated: classroom Reality Orientation, where people have a half-hour session daily; and ward-based 24-hour Reality Orientation, where cues in the environment and contacts with staff throughout the 24 hours are used to reinforce orientation. It appears that classroom Reality Orientation can improve cognitive functioning, but that the 24-hour ward orientation training may in addition improve behaviour (Hanley et al, 1981).

The family

Any change in relationships requires adjustment. It can be painful to see a relative or friend change mentally and deteriorate. It can be a frustrating experience trying to communicate with a relative who fails to understand. It may be embarrassing or even offensive to have to wash and clean up after an incontinent parent. Guilt at not being able to cope with an elderly parent, the time spent away from one's own children and guilt at changing emotions are all difficult to deal with. The move into permanent institutional care and eventual death are further stresses.

How best can we help with these problems? Individual counselling is aimed at allowing relatives to speak about both the acceptable feelings that they experience and the unacceptable, including the dreadful thoughts and feelings that so commonly occur in these situations, but which seem so alien and terrible to those experiencing them for the first time. The feelings of hate, anger, despair, even the thought that the old person would be better off dead. The family are grieving for the loss of the healthy person that they knew. Like any grief, it may be intense and painful. The family must be helped to see that this is a normal, healthy reaction to a distressing change in their life and be helped through this difficult period.

Sometimes, it is difficult for relatives to understand why the aggressive, demanding and frustrating old person that caused them so much difficulty and distress is apparently so well behaved and easily managed by the hospital staff. They may take this as a personal failure on their part. The staff must help them to understand that it is often easier to cope with troublesome people who are not relatives and with whom one does not have the same emotional ties. Secondly, the staff are only in contact with the patient for a maximum of an eight-hour shift, and often this is shared between a number of staff. The relative has been in contact with the old person often for 24 hours out of 24. No wonder they found it difficult.

Relatives' groups

Individual counselling of relatives is always useful, but it is helpful for them to meet others in the 'same boat'. It is good to know that the problems, feelings and experiences that seemed so unique to them, are in fact shared by others.

Voluntary support groups such as the Alzheimer's Disease Society provide this sort of support as well as education, advice and fund raising activities for research.

Problem behaviour

The behaviour often described as being most difficult for the family to cope with is the restlessness, repetitive questions or actions, wandering and incontinence of the elderly patient. Other problem behaviours include dangerousness, violence, drinking, suicidal actions and Capgras syndrome (which will be described below).

Major tranquillisers (see Ch. 6) may reduce agitation, aggression and, given at night, may help sleep to occur at the normal time. The old person should not be permitted to sleep during the day as this will reduce the amount of sleep required at night. Incontinence may be helped by a variety of devices, pads and waterproof garments, but the development of a regular routine and clear labelling of toilet doors will undoubtedly be of help.

Dangerous behaviour, such as not lighting the gas cooker reliably, or forgetting about burning cigarette ends, is a constant source of concern for relatives and neighbours. Old cookers and heaters should be replaced by modern appliances with built-in safety devices. The hazards of smoking may be restricted by limiting smoking to when another person is present or the installation of a relatively cheap battery-operated smoke alarm.

The Capgras syndrome is a not-uncommon symptom of brain failure. The old person becomes convinced that his relatives have been replaced by people who are only pretending to be relatives. He sees these bogus relatives as evil and will address all manner of dreadful and hurtful remarks to them. It is very difficult for the family to cope, especially if they do not recognise that this is part of the illness and not addressed at them personally. Unfortunately, there is no specific treatment for this state of affairs and considerable support and explanation must be given to the family.

Suicide

The old, especially those who are lonely and have experienced recent loss, are at increased risk of suicide. The risk is especially high during the year following the loss of a spouse, in all divorced and widowed people and those with physical illness. Alcohol abuse and lack of social ties are also risk factors.

Suicide in the old, as with all age groups, is closely associated with depressive illness and the survivor of any suicidal behaviour should be carefully screened for depression which, if present, should be actively treated.

Capacity to manage affairs

Deterioration may render a person quite incapable of understanding and managing financial or legal affairs. Thus, a patient may get into financial difficulties through incompetence or he may be at risk of exploitation. In order to protect the muddled old person, it may be necessary for someone else to take over the management of his affairs. In many cases, this will be a near relative to whom the old person will give power of attorney, that is, the old person voluntarily hands over control of his affairs to relatives. This process assumes that the elderly person is capable of understanding what this means.

In other cases, where there is no suitable relative or where the old person is unable to give consent, a lawyer may be appointed. This requires medical evidence that the individual is incapable, through illness, of managing his affairs.

These legal procedures are by no means a recent innovation, but date back to ancient Greece. Sophocles' son applied to the Court for the appointment of a 'Committee of the Person' on the grounds that, owing to old age, his father was unable to manage his affairs. Sophocles is supposed to have said the following to the Court: 'If I am Sophocles, I am not beside myself; if I am beside myself, I am not Sophocles'.

Testamentary capacity

If an old person, especially with some degree of confusion or memory disturbance, is to make a new will, it is advisable to obtain a medical opinion as to the old person's ability to understand and know what he is doing. This will avoid argument when eventually the will comes to be read.

OTHER PSYCHIATRIC DISORDERS IN THE ELDERLY

Any of the disorders of earlier life may continue into old age or return then. Thus, neuroses and personality disorders, which always manifest themselves earlier in life may cause problems into old age but will never appear for the first time at that stage.

Depressive illness (manic depressive illness:—depressed type, endogenous depression).

Depressive illness is a condition of middle to old age. In the elderly, agitation and delusions may be prominent, leading to a failure to eat and drink and a rapid deterioration of physical health. Electroconvulsive therapy (E.C.T.) probably has a more rapid onset of action than antidepressants and is also safer than drugs in this elderly group of patients.

Common delusions in the elderly:

delusion	*example*
paranoid	conviction that food and water are poisoned
guilt	conviction that the old person has committed a crime or does not deserve food, etc.
poverty	unable to pay for food or keep
nihilistic	conviction that one's insides are rotting away, etc.

Pseudo-dementia

This occurs occasionally in severely depressed old people. Over a relatively short period of time, the old person changes from being normal to appearing quite demented: confused, forgetful, unable to grasp what is happening about him. The clues to the diagnosis are the rapidity of change, which is far faster than is usual for chronic brain failure; and a past history of depression or of other symptoms and signs suggestive of depression such as early morning wakening or diurnal mood variation.

In cases of doubt, a sodium amytal interview may be useful. An interview conducted after the administration of sodium amytal either intravenously or by mouth may enable a patient suffering from depressive pseudo-dementia to communicate better or to talk about worries or delusions, whereas there will be no change in the truly demented person. Once identified, the depression should be treated.

Acute brain failure (acute confusional state, delirium)

This always occurs secondary to some other condition. Common causes are acute physical illness such as pneumonia or urinary tract infections, prescribed medication, especially sleeping tablets and tranquillisers, withdrawal from alcohol or drugs and metabolic conditions such as uncontrolled diabetes.

The patient is confused, has clouding of consciousness and may hallucinate (usually visually) or misinterpret what is happening about him (illusions). The patient appears anxious, perplexed and frightened and this is usually worse at night. The treatment is of the underlying cause. During the acute phase, the patient may be helped by being nursed in quiet, well lit surroundings with the minimum of staff changes.

Paraphrenia

The paranoid psychosis of old age, has a variable response to treatment with major tranquillisers. After an adequate trial, if no improvement is seen, the drugs should be withdrawn.

Many old people can live comfortably in the community harbouring many strange ideas as long as they can be encouraged only to talk about them to the caring staff and not to bother neighbours, friends and the police. Intellectual functioning and memory are not affected by this illness.

Mrs X, a 70-year-old widow, became convinced that local policemen visited her nightly and sexually assaulted her with their truncheons. Her frequent complaints to the neighbours and the local police led to demands for action. Medication made no difference to her delusions. Slowly, over a period of time, a community psychiatric nurse gained the confidence of Mrs X. She agreed to save all her worries until the weekly visit by the nurse. Now, as she does not talk about the delusions, which persist, she is again an acceptable member of the local community.

Unidentified physical illness

Psychological or physical change in an old person should not automatically be attributed to a psychiatric disorder just because no obvious physical illness has been noted. There must be a full psychiatric assessment with sufficient grounds to justify a positive psychiatric diagnosis, not just the absence of obvious physical illness. In any case of doubt, routine physical screening tests should be carried out including full physical examination, routine haematology including ESR, liver function tests, thyroxine (T_4), urinalysis, and plain chest and skull X-rays. Further specific tests may be indicated.

DEATH, DYING AND BEREAVEMENT

Thoughts of death tend to increase with age and, in general, most old people come to terms with and accept the inevitability of their own death and the death of elderly friends and relatives. In fact, many lonely old people, especially those with chronic physical disorders, look upon death as a welcome relief. Despite these attitudes, death will bring a period of grief, bereavement and adjustment to the new situation.

Lindemann, in his classic study of grief, pointed out that grief is a normal, healthy response to a distressing situation. Although the detailed manifestations of grief will vary from person to person depending on the circumstances, everyone passes through the three phases of grief (See below).

The stages of grief:

Stage 1 shock, numbness, disbelief, lasts for a few hours to a few days.

Stage 2 full grieving, ruminations about the death and the dead person, tearful, socially withdrawn, loss of appetite, difficulty sleeping, frequent anger and guilt, a need to talk about the dead person, separation anxiety (the anxiety associated with being left alone) and recurrent grief pangs.

Stage 3 resolution, accepting the death, separating from the dead person, becoming able to make new relationships and plans without devaluing the dead person.

Lindemann suggested that appropriate help at times of crisis such as grief could reduce the incidence of pathology. It is hoped that by promoting healthy grieving, fewer people will go on to develop abnormally prolonged grief reactions or even mental illness.

Simple guidelines to promote healthy grieving

These simple measures may be applied by the staff and, better still, can be taught to the relatives of the bereaved. The bereaved person: (1) must be allowed/encouraged to talk about the dead person and to express their grief without embarrassment and without the fear that others will not be able to cope with this show of emotion; (2) must be encouraged to see grief as a normal healthy response which will not be helped (and almost certainly will be hindered) by the use of minor tranquillisers or anti-depressants; (3) must understand that the grieving is a necessary part of the process of coming to terms with what has happened in their life; (4) many bereaved people are terrified that they are 'going crazy' because of the bizarre experiences following the death. Yet the majority will feel that they see, hear or feel the presence of the dead person during the few weeks after the death. They are often terrified to mention this to even their closest friends. They may be greatly relieved to be asked if they have had any of these experiences and to be told that they are very common and normal.

The relatives must be encouraged to follow these guidelines and especially not to try to distract the bereaved person from his grief. With the best of intentions relatives try to talk about anything but the death and to suggest an immediate move of house or a holiday to make the person less distressed. Attempts to deny the impact of death may leave the bereaved unable to express the appropriate emotion.

Mr G was on holiday with his wife in a remote Third World country when she was suddenly taken ill and died. For the next few days, he was totally occupied with completing the complex arrangements to register his wife's death and organise her cremation prior to his return to Britain. He was surprised to note that he felt and showed no emotion at his wife's death. It was only three months later when, waking out of a sleep in front of the television, he thought he heard his wife moving about the house. Almost immediately, he became aware that this was impossible and that she was dead. For the first time, he felt the desolation and distress and wept. This delayed grief reaction could perhaps have been prevented if there had been someone with whom he could have shared his distress at the time of the event.

Dying

It is not only bereaved relatives who experience grief but also the dying. They are grieving for loss of health, loss of life and loss of a future. The process is very similar to the grief experienced by relatives and they must be allowed, if they wish, to talk about and freely express these emotions. Frequently, they are encouraged not to show emotion and are praised by medical staff and relatives alike for having a 'stiff upper lip' and coping so well with the knowledge of their terminal illness. This manoeuvre to prevent the show of emotion is often to help the relatives and staff cope at the expense of the dying person.

The dying must be given time and opportunity to talk about what is happening to them. This does not mean being asked on a ward round whether they want to talk about the future but a sensitive counselling approach with privacy and time.

Death and the clinical team

The impact that the death of a patient has on members of the clinical team is often underestimated, particularly where the patient is very well known to the staff or where the death is sudden or in some other way traumatic such as suicide or a painful cancer. The team must have a built-in opportunity to discuss the emotional impact of such an event at a regular team meeting or sensitivity meeting. Also, all team members should be sensitive to the impact such an event has on themselves and on individual team members who might need particular support at that time.

PROBLEMS OF WORKING WITH THE ELDERLY

Fortunately, a large number of staff positively enjoy working with elderly patients. However, this is by no means universal. The Group for the Advancement of Psychiatry (1971) identified several reasons why many people are reluctant to deal with the elderly. The main points of this report may prove useful in team discussion and in sensitivity meetings.

The main findings are:

(1) the aged stimulate the therapist's (helper's) fears about his own old age;

(2) they arouse conflicts about his own relationships with parental figures;

(3) the therapist believes he has nothing useful to offer old people because he believes they cannot change their behaviour or that their problems are all due to untreatable organic brain disease;

(4) The therapist believes that his skills will be wasted if he works with the aged because they are near death and not really deserving of attention;

(5) the therapist's colleagues may be contemptuous of his efforts on behalf of aged patients.

CONCLUSIONS

This chapter has not attempted to provide a comprehensive review of rehabilitation with elderly patients. It has focussed on the problems of normal ageing in order to help identify what is due to illness and what is an accepted part of normal ageing. Attention should also be drawn to the dangers inherent in treating old people. In particular, an over-zealous attempt to treat all physical illnesses may lead to a poorer quality of life due to drug side-effects, especially since old people are more sensitive to medication. It is worth remembering Napoleon's statement, 'I do not want two diseases— one nature-made, one doctor-made.' (Napoleon Bonaparte, 1820).

REFERENCES

Cumming E, Henry W E 1961 Growing old. Basic Books, New York
DHSS 1982 Social trends No. 12. HMSO, London
Group for the Advancement of Psychiatry 1971 The aged and community mental health. Mental Health Materials Center, New York
Hanley I G, Mc Guire R J, Boyd W D 1981 Reality orientation and dementia: a controlled trial of two approaches. British Journal of Psychiatry 138: 10–14

Kinsey A S, Pomeroy W B, Martin C R 1948 Sexual behaviour in the human male. Saunders, Philadelphia

Lindemann E 1944 Symptomatology and management of acute grief. American Journal of Psychiatry 101:141

Maddox G L 1963 Activity—morale: a longitudinal study of selected elderly subjects. Social Forces 42:195

Masters W H, Johnson V E 1970 Human sexual inadequacy. Little Brown, Boston

Moyes I 1980 The psychiatry of old age. S, K & F Publications, London

World Health Organization 1983 The elderly in eleven countries. A sociomedical study. Public Health in Europe No. 21. WHO, Geneva

Life is not a matter of holding good cards, but of playing a poor hand well.

Robert Louis Stevenson

13

Physical disability

Clephane Hume

It is generally accepted, but not always remembered, that a patient's psychological state will influence his recovery. A patient who is psychologically healthy yet severely physically disabled may well reach a higher level of independence than his fellow patient who is poorly motivated due to psychological problems. Adjustment to, and acceptance of disability are vital if recovery and independence are to be achieved. The concept of handicap in the context of psychiatric illness is described in Chapter 2. The same ideas can be applied to physical disorders; those disabilities which arise as part of the illness and the secondary handicaps which are a result of having been ill (their own or other people's reactions to the illness). But this must be seen in the context of the individual. The level of handicap may be very different from the level of impairment (the measureable physical disability). A minor impairment, such as stiffness in one finger caused by arthritis, could put an end to the career of a concert pianist. An office worker, with a similar level of impairment, might not consider himself to be disabled in any way.

THE COPING PROCESS

The adjustment to physical disability has been described by

209

Wright (1960), Roessler and Bolton (1978), and Power and Dell Orto (1980). The sequence of psychological events which constitutes the coping process has been described by Falek (1984). The coping process after loss of health or physical ability is similar to the reaction to other major losses such as bereavement.

The stages of coping are:
— Denial
— Anxiety and searching
— Anger
— Depression
— Resolution.

Denial

The initial reaction to physical injury or diagnosis of a disabling condition is numbness and shock. This may be accompanied by disbelief and an immediate refusal to accept that life will be in any way changed. The immediate appearance of denial cushions the individual against the full implications of the event by allowing him to ignore the painful aspects of the situation. Gradually the stage of denial is replaced by a full realisation of the situation and its implications.

It is important to remember that during the denial phase the patient is unable to discuss fully his situation. Even if he seems to be reacting in a mature and rational manner (with a 'stiff upper lip') he will not be in a position to make reasonable decisions about his future or rehabilitation plans.

Awaiting surgical amputation of his dominant arm, Sandy resisted all attempts to develop the use of his other arm. He could see no reason to do so despite the careful explanations he was given. Because of denial he was unable to move on to consider the significance of this situation.

Anxiety and searching

As denial recedes, the gradual realisation that the injury or illness is continuing leads to anxiety and a search for an explanation. 'Why has this happened to me?' 'What have I done to deserve this?' Depending upon the level of anxiety it is possible to initiate discussions regarding future management.

Alternatively, the searching may be continued until all possibilities are exhausted in a vain attempt to find a cure rather than accept the situation.

Bill, realising that he had a hemiparesis that could not be cured by conventional medicine, consulted a herbalist, an acupuncturist and a faith healer. Clutching at any new idea which offered hope, only as each one was eliminated, did he begin to move towards the third stage of the adjustment process.

Anger

This can prove very distressing for patient, relatives, friends and, not least, those involved in treatment. The patient may feel that if only the doctors had cared for him a little more then they would have tried harder to cure him. He may feel resentful of the contact he has with all members of the team. A distressing manifestation of anger for the believer is the experience of anger with God. 'How can I believe in a God who does this to me?' Family members may be made to feel that, if only they had insisted on medical treatment earlier or had in some other way intervened, the physical handicap might have been avoided. In some cases the anger is directed towards the self, resulting in guilt and depression.

Depression

Depression and mourning indicate that the individual is working through the stages of coping. He has accepted that the disability exists and that his earlier attempts at altering the situation have been unsuccessful. He grieves for the loss of health, loss of function and status, and for the opportunities that will be denied him. He may ruminate on his predicament, becoming withdrawn and uncommunicative. His misery and lack of drive may interfere with his treatment programme.

Resolution

Finally the person enters a stage of resolution. Although grief pangs will occur from time to time, the separation from his old life and earlier aspirations and a readiness to consider the future as a handicapped person show that the mourning process has been accomplished. Now he has accepted that he is handicapped, he is ready to learn to live with the disability and to learn ways of coping which will allow him to be as independent as possible. The rehabilitation process is under way.

FACTORS AFFECTING ADJUSTMENT

Virtually everybody confronted with the prospect of physical disability will experience these reactions to their handicap. As with other forms of mourning the pattern, although sticking to the recognised stages, will be very variable. Reactions will be coloured by the individual's personality and coping patterns in response to earlier crises as well as to the onset of the problem and its severity.

The disability may be acquired suddenly and traumatically (paraplegia following a diving accident, a limb severed in a traffic accident) or may be insidious in onset and progressively disabling (multiple sclerosis, rheumatoid arthritis). The illness may be life-threatening (renal failure maintained by dialysis) or terminal (carcinoma). The adjustment to terminal illness has been described by Elizabeth Kübler Ross (1970).

Congenital disability, such as spina bifida, probably requires more adjustment from the family than the child himself. Although it may be true that people will not mourn the loss of an ability which they never possessed, a sense of lack and of being different from other will be learned from the attitudes of the people they meet in their daily lives.

In addition to having to cope with the initial guilt of 'producing a disabled child', the parents will have to live with the social, emotional and financial problems of handicap. It has been suggested that a handicapped child means a handicapped family. The restrictions which the disability imposes on the family members in terms of mobility, holidays, social activities or financial constraints affect the whole family. Siblings may feel resentful or neglected and their opportunities may be restricted by the need to take a share in caring for the disabled family member.

At an early stage, the disabled child may wonder, like some

of the thalidomide children, when his disability will go away. 'When will my arms grow?' 'When will my legs be strong enough to walk on?'

All these reactions are normal. Rehabilitation staff should understand that as these reactions are normal and healthy they should be expressed and are not to be ignored or avoided in a conspiracy of silence.

ADJUSTMENT PROBLEMS

For some, the process of adjustment will be incomplete. The severity of the condition, the patient's personality, his social circumstances or lack of support may prevent him from fully working through all stages of the coping process.

Mild or transient anxiety, depression and hostility can be regarded as normal responses to the circumstances in which the disabled person finds himself. Prolonged or severe reactions create difficulties which may require specific intervention.

Anxiety may be made worse if the patient does not fully understand what is going on around him; complicated medical equipment, tests, and fears and apprehensions about the future. Simple explanations will usually be reassuring, but if not, his anxiety may grow out of proportion to the reality of the situation. An example is the person who is terrified that minor exertion will precipitate another heart attack and who therefore avoids any exercise.

Depression may cause the individual to withdraw and to see everything in a very negative light. He views active therapy as a useless exercise. When all seems hopeless, what is the point?

When anger and resentment predominate, the patient becomes critical, abusive and demanding of staff. Other patients will avoid him as may staff, especially the less experienced who may take his comments personally.

The psychological stress of handicap may precipitate a major psychiatric illness (usually depressive illness or paranoid psychosis). Medication, or its withdrawal, may cause an acute organic confusional state. Staff must be vigilant in their assessment of the patient's stage of coping. Has the depression of the coping process turned into a depressive illness requiring specific treatment? Prevention of the additional handicaps of institutionalisation should be pursued, particularly where the hospital stay is likely to be prolonged. While psychological defences such as denial are part of the healthy coping process, prolonged use of the defence mechanism with an inability to pass on to the next stage of the coping process may prevent resolution occuring and hinder the rehabilitation programme.

The growing sub-speciality of liaison psychiatry should lead to an increased awareness of the psychological factors associated with physical illness and handicap, and hopefully earlier referral for specialist help.

PROBLEMS ENCOUNTERED DURING REHABILITATION

Acceptance of disability is the first important step in the rehabilitation process. Having dealt with his own emotional reactions and learned to cope with his physical limitations, the patient has to contend with the barriers to integration imposed by society, and the reaction of his family and friends.

Barriers to integration

Physical barriers such as restricted access to buildings, transport and general restriction on mobility are obvious. More insidious are the psychological barriers. Some disabilities may force people into having social contact mainly with similarly affected people because of either mobility problems or the need for assistance. Special transport is expensive and since many handicapped people will not be working, and are relying on state benefits, they may have very limited opportunity to leave the house.

For people who have 'hidden' or 'invisible' disabilities, there is the added problem of appearing 'normal' and yet not behaving as expected. It may not be obvious that someone is partially sighted and people do not look deaf. (Modern hearing aids may be unhelpfully discreet.) Speech problems may be immediately apparent, while dietary restrictions may not be noticed for some time if the sufferer is adept at coping.

The greatest of all barriers is, however, the attitude of society. Rejection or revulsion, curiosity, patronising behaviour, or smothering help all severely hamper the disabled person's integration. 'Does he take sugar?' has become a well known phrase in the United Kingdom following a radio programme with that title. But the problems behind the question are still not fully understood by the general public, despite education and public relations exercises by a wide number of people and organisations. The widely publicised 'International year of the disabled' (1981) did much to draw the public's attention to the difficulties faced by the disabled, but with the ending of the year the focus of public attention shifted elsewhere. (An obvious disability may have some compensations.)

Psychosocial problems

Physical handicap is a stigma (Goffman, 1964) and may lead to the sufferer being ostracised.

Within the family there will be changes in roles and therefore in status (Ch. 10). The husband who has been breadwinner, do-it-yourself handyman and financial administrator may find his wife taking over all these roles. His role as father may be restricted by his inability to enjoy physical recreation with his children while his role as husband may be altered by difficulty in achieving a mutually satisfactory sexual relationship with his wife. He may feel that his status within the family has been devalued.

Obviously, this is the blackest side of the picture, but it nevertheless illustrates some of the obstacles. The degree of handicap and pre-existing family relationships will influence which problems arise.

Difficulties may also occur for the patient and his family at other levels. The move to accomodation providing easier access may entail the whole family coping with a new neighbourhood, neighbours and a change of school for the children. Friends who have conscientiously visited the patient in hospital may assume that on his return home they can withdraw their attention. It can be a hindrance and embarrassment to take a disabled person on social outings or holidays and although there may be no malicious intent, the individual may find himself excluded. All these factors may lead to enforced isolation and loneliness.

PHYSICAL CONDITIONS PRODUCING PSYCHIATRIC SYMPTOMS

Certain physical illnesses may present with psychiatric symptoms (Table 13.1).

Table 13.1 Some psychiatric symptoms related to physical disorders

Physical condition		Psychiatric symptoms
endocrine	thyrotoxicosis	anxiety, overactivity
	myxoedema	depression, dementia
	pituitary	euphoria, depression
	diabetes	confusion
infections	virus e.g. influenza and mononucleosis (glandular fever)	depression (may be profound)
	infection causing high temperature	confusion (delirium)
nervous system	tumour	confusion
	multiple sclerosis	euphoria, depression
	head injury	personality change, dementia
cardio vascular	heart failure	confusion, paranoia, memory disturbance
drugs and alcohol	alcohol withdrawal	DTs (confusion)
	alcohol addiction	dementia, recent memory disturbance
prescribed drugs	methyl dopa	profound depression
	steroids	euphoria, confusion, paranoia
illegal drugs		psychosis, withdrawal, confusion

In all cases the quality of life, and benefits of treatment must be weighed against the restrictions imposed on the individual and undesirable effects of treatment. 'Treatment at all costs' may lead to a very poor quality of life.

Sensory deficits, especially deafness and blindness, which cut people off from the world around them, may be associated with paranoia as communication is only partially heard and misinterpreted.

The special needs of young chronically disabled patients may be hard to meet. These patients may lack the mobility, communication or social skills which are required for social relationships to develop. Sensitive help is required to encourage normal social contact with others. Clubs such as PHAB (physically handicapped and able bodied) may sound contrived, but can provide fun and participation in a range of activities.

Sexual needs may be more difficult to deal with because of staff attitudes: 'It isn't nice', 'What would happen if the papers heard about it?' The frustration of being in close proximity with others to whom the patient feels attracted but without the privacy in which to have a closer relationship may be considerable. Even if sexual intercourse is not physically possible or is taboo within the institution, privacy may afford a degree of closeness of physical contact which can lead to a mutually satisfying relationship. It might be helpful to remember that amongst the general public in British, sexual relationships outside marriage and homosexual relationships are commonly accepted. Rehabilitation staff must reflect society.

PSYCHIATRIC PROBLEMS CONTRIBUTING TO PHYSICAL ILLNESS

Eating disorders and addictions may cause major physical disorder. The gross malnutrition resulting from severe anorexia nervosa will produce widespread physiological changes. In extreme cases death or permanent impairment (e.g. renal failure) will occur.

Alcohol abuse and the associated vitamin deficiency produce a variety of neurological changes including sensory impairment, recent memory impairment and dementia. Alcoholics are prone to accidental injury and gastro-intestinal disorders (gastritis, ulcers, liver failure).

Intravenous drug abusers are at high risk of physical illness:

hepatitis from sharing needles, septicaemia from faculty injection technique and thrombosis from the injection of 'non injectable' substances. As more veins become thrombosed and therefore impossible to use, the addict may resort to the large, but hidden blood vessels in the groin (femoral vein) with disastrous results. Infection, thrombosis or damage to the femoral artery may lead to gangrene and the need for amputation of the leg. In addition to the problems of overdose, drug-induced psychosis and withdrawal states for the addict, attention has recently focussed on the effect of addiction on the developing fetus and the neonatal withdrawal syndrome.

Some severely psychotic patients are at risk of self-harm in response to hallucinations or delusions. Terry, who suffered from schizophrenia, was ordered by his 'voices' to throw himself from a railway bridge. David cut off his arm because he regarded it as housing all the 'evil' in his body and had great difficulty in accepting and using a prosthesis. Self-castration and other mutilating acts may accompany sexual delusions.

But it is not only psychotic people who damage themselves. Mary, who had an impulsive and antisocial personality, swallowed cutlery and a variety of other objects with such frequency that she received a near-injurious dose of radiation from all the X-rays taken. People who, under the influence of alcohol, drugs or distress, jump from high buildings may sustain multiple fractures. Their progress may depend a lot on their mental state and personality. Management of patients who sustain major physical injuries may not be possible within a psychiatric hospital but the psychiatric team should endeavour to maintain close contact with the medical team as well as with their patient.

MANAGEMENT OF PSYCHOLOGICAL PROBLEMS IN PHYSICAL REHABILITATION

Abnormal psychological difficulties can be minimised, if not actually prevented, by the attitudes of the rehabilitation team. Essentially it is a matter of time, openness, accurate information, honesty and encouragement for the patient to express worries and fears, however embarrassing or ridiculous.

It is easy to forget how strange and frightening most hospitals are. The patient requires straightforward information and non-technical explanations. If patients feel that they will not be regarded as stupid if they ask apparently trivial questions, that in itself is reassuring.

Patients are often reluctant to raise emotionally loaded or embarrassing questions. Staff must learn to broach these topics in a sensitive but matter-of-fact way when a suitable opportunity presents itself, and be sensitive to any hints the patient gives. This applies particularly to marital and sexual problems. Simple information may be enough, but further counselling may be required.

The patient may be frightened by side-effects of medication. While explanation may help, it is preferable to warn patients of possible side-effects in advance. Information will not make the side-effects any fewer, but knowing the cause may make them more tolerable.

Honesty is essential. An honest appraisal of the patient's prognosis may be difficult for everyone to face and difficult to give, but unrealistic expectations and false hopes only lead to disappointment and lack of trust. It is usually possible to give an honest account without totally destroying hope.

It is often easier for staff if patients do not express the anger, frustration or distress they feel. Staff may, quite unconsciously, encourage and reinforce stoicism and avoid any show of emotion. It is much healthier for the patient to express the feelings he has, however difficult for the staff.

Searching for a miracle cure may prevent the patient from accepting his situation. Other coping mechanisms that outlive their usefulness may be equally detrimental. The old adage 'take one day at a time' may be appropriate for the acute phase of coping, but quite inappropriate when longer-term plans are being made. Religious faith may be a help and comfort to some patients, enabling them to come to terms with their situation as it is 'God's will'. Other religious people will be distressed by their loss of faith when faced with the catastrophe. 'How could God do this to me?' Whatever the team members' own religious views, it behoves them to be empathetic and to respect the patient's view.

Voluntary self-help organisations may provide considerable

support. Some examples of organisations operating in the United Kingdom are the Spinal Injuries Association, Headway (head injuries) or the Parkinson's Disease Society. They provide information and advice and may have resources which enable them to provide social activities or sheltered work. Special housing or holidays may also be available and these provide support for relatives and patients alike.

Some organisations, e.g. D.I.G. (Disablement Income Group) act as a pressure group, campaigning for the needs of the disabled and for suitable provision.

Relationships between professionals and voluntary groups are very variable, but it is worth remembering that a fellow sufferer may be able to communicate with and provide very valuable support for a patient. There are two other aspects of management: the understanding of the needs of different cultures, particularly minority ethnic groups, and the use of health education and self-help techniques.

The rehabilitation team should be familiar with immigrant groups within their locality and should adapt their approach according to needs. If, for example, it is regarded as being the family's responsibility to care for their disabled relative or to make decisions about his future, this has obvious implications for rehabilitation. The team should know where to obtain help and advice, including interpretation if this is required.

Health education is already used in the prevention of problems, and awareness of relaxation techniques and yoga has led to individuals practising them. The reduction in stress may be considerable. A recent innovation has been the introduction of assertiveness training for cardiac patients. By learning to identify different styles of behaviour, people can modify their own responses and reduce stress in interpersonal relationships.

Group discussion may be an idea which seems unacceptable to people whose disabilities are primarily physical. However, modern trends do lean towards more self-examination and self-disclosure than has formerly been allowable, and a regular problem-sharing group is worthy of consideration.

CONCLUSION

There is considerable overlap between physical and psychiatric disorder. It is easy for psychiatric staff to be critical of the treatment of physical illness without any apparent recognition of the psychological sequelae. But it is salutary to remember that patients with psychiatric symptoms may well be suffering from an unrecognised physical disorder.

REFERENCES

Falek A 1984 Sequential aspects of the coping process. In: Emery A E H, Pullen I M Psychological aspects of genetic counselling. Academic Press, London, p 23–36
Gelder M, Gath D H, Mayou R 1983 Oxford textbook of psychiatry. Oxford University Press, Oxford
Goffman E 1968 Stigma. Notes of the management of spoiled identity. Penguin, Harmondsworth
Grellier D 1984 Physical dysfunction. In: Willson M Occupational therapy in short term psychiatry. Churchill Livingstone, Edinburgh.
Kübler Ross E 1970 On death and dying. Social Science Paperbacks, Tavistock, London
Power P W, Dell Orto A E 1980 The role of the family in the rehabilitation of the physically disabled. University Park Press, Baltimore
Pullen I M 1984 Physical handicap. In: Emery A E, Pullen I M Psychological aspects of genetic counselling. Academic Press, London, p 107–124
Roessler R, Bolton B 1978 Psychosocial adjustment to disability. University Park Press, Baltimore
Shakespeare R 1975 The psychology of handicap. Methuen, Essential Psychology, London
Wright B 1983 Physical disability, a psychological approach, 2nd edn. Harper Row, London
Zealley A 1983 Psychiatry in general medicine. In: Kendell R, Zealley A (eds) Companion to psychiatric studies, 3rd edn. Churchill Livingstone, Edinburgh p 557

If you'll believe in me, I'll believe in you.

Lewis Carroll *Through the Looking-Glass*

14

The future

Clephane Hume and Ian Pullen

Rehabilitation is a relatively young branch of psychiatry. Within its short life there have been many changes including the move from compulsory to voluntary admissions, the introduction of effective treatments, the scientific evaluation of drug and social therapies, and the return of many patients to the community. But what for the future? Some changes are inevitable and easy to predict: others are more speculative.

Rehabilitation teams must be flexible and accept change. Already the patient population has changed. In Britain, the original longterm patients have been resettled and younger patients are being discharged earlier. The focus of rehabilitation is moving away from deinstitutionalisation towards prevention of dependence, and maintenance in the community. Increased emphasis is being placed on preventive work with families.

The trend towards community care will continue. Already in England and Wales plans are underway to close whole hospitals. The staff are being asked to plan the community facilities that will be required in order to care for discharged patients. With the continuing economic recession there is a danger that not all of the necessary facilities will be provided and there will be a reduction in services.

Not all of the predictions are so gloomy. Experimental

alternatives to hospital care will continue to be investigated. The plan to replace longstay wards by housing schemes within the hospital grounds (proposed for Friern Barnet hospital in North London) or in different parts of the city (Oslo) are two such examples.

The increased emphasis placed on research in biological psychiatry may lead us to expect progress in the under-standing of illnesses such as schizophrenia and hence new treatments. Unfortunately this seems unlikely to happen. The introduction of effective drug treatments occurred, not as the result of biological research, but from close observation of the effects of drugs being used for other conditions, mistaken theories or serendipity.

Technology will play an increasing part in management and treatment, whether for administrative purposes or for direct therapy. The availability of mental health education programs for use on home computers does not seem too remote a possibility.

Service industries, including the health and social services, are expensive to run. In Britain, for purely financial reasons, there has been a reduction in the number of social workers and nurses. This trend seems set to continue. Therefore rehabilitation services must become more efficient, and be seen to be cost effective. Rather than replace the multi-disci-plinary approach to assessment by a medical or nursing assessment, it may be necessary to work in a different way with more role blurring, but taking care to avoid duplication. To this end, how much of a nurse's, a social worker's or a doctor's training is used from day to day in rehabilitation? Many of the skills are acquired only after starting to work in the speciality. Perhaps we shall see the development of a Mental Health Professional or a Rehabilitation Worker with training more pertinent to the work.

The most exciting development is likely to take place over the next three to four years. The discovery of a genetic marker for Huntington's disease is likely to be followed by the intro-duction of predictive tests for schizophrenia, Alzheimer's disease, manic-depressive illness and other inherited conditions.

Other predictions will depend on government decisions. At present it looks as though unemployment, drug abuse, alcoholism and head injuries will continue to increase. All could be reduced by the right policies. Perhaps the community will at last become more aware and more responsive to the needs of people with psychiatric illness so that the attitudes of society are more positive and self-help facilities are more acceptable. Health education in the mental health field may be regarded by some as a luxury but if the future of our communities is at stake it seems a worthwhile investment. City planners, defence experts and government officials can all help to reduce stress. Indeed we can all contribute. Prevention, after all, is better than cure.

Rehabilitation is a young speciality. Much interest lies in the fact that it is still developing. Probably the most exciting developments will be those that no one has yet even thought of!

Index

225